Drama and Healing
The Roots of Drama Therapy

Roger Grainger

Jessica Kingsley Publishers

London and Bristol, Pennsylvania

First published in hardback in the United Kingdom in 1990 by
Jessica Kingsley Publishers Ltd
116 Pentonville Road
London N1 9JB, England
and
1900 Frost Road, Suite 101
Bristol, PA 19007, U S A

First published in paperback in 1995

Library of Congress Cataloging in Publication Data
A CIP catalogue record for this book is available from the Library of Congress

British Library Cataloguing in Publication Data
A CIP catalogue record for this book is available from the British Library

ISBN 1-85302-337-X

Printed and Bound in Great Britain by
Athenaeum Press, Gateshead, Tyne and Wear

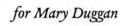

for Mary Duggan

Contents

Introduction 9

Part I Roots

Chapter 1 Drama as Involvement 17

Chapter 2 The Healing Symbol 30

Chapter 3 Drama and Depression 40

Chapter 4 Drama and Schizophrenia 53

Part II Process

Chapter 5 Approaches to Drama Therapy 71

Chapter 6 Some of the Cast 83

Chapter 7 Capturing the Image 99

Chapter 8 Drama Therapy and Ritual 118

Appendix 1 The use of drama therapy in
the treatment of thought disorder 133

Appendix 2 Instructions for administering
the grid test of thought disorder 142

Appendix 3 Programme of BAC National Conference, 1989 144

Bibliography 145

Glossary 149

Index 151

Introduction

This book is mainly concerned with drama therapy. However it did not seem either reasonable or possible to deal at all adequately with the therapeutic application of drama without looking first of all at the nature of the art form itself, in order to 'set the scene' for a consideration of what it is that makes drama therapy a healing experience for psychologically disturbed people.

The first part of the book, Chapters 1 to 4, starts out by investigating the therapeutic origins of theatre before moving on to the part played by drama in psychological maturation. Important in itself, this serves to introduce a more focused consideration of alienated psychological states which distort human relationship. Chapters 3 and 4 concern depression, thought disorder and schizophrenia. An investigation of the use of drama therapy in the treatment of thought disorder, carried out as part of a CNAA research project, revealed a heightened degree of cognitive clarity to be communicable through dramatic experience, a finding which gave substance to the ideas put forward in the earlier part of the book. Drama therapy aims at providing an environment which is emotionally secure and structurally identifiable, in which role relationships are clearly defined and epistemological categories easily distinguished. Not only those diagnosed as schizophrenic, but depressed people too benefit from an approach which is not any kind of imitation of life but a participation in the essential processes of human experience, a way of communicating the truth about the relationship between self and other upon which flexibility and definition of thought and feeling depend. Part 2, then, is concerned with the drama therapy *experience*.

Because drama has an effect on the way in which we make our own personal sense out of our environment of people and things, I have used George Kelly's Personal Construct Theory as a way of ordering my own thoughts throughout the book. (Most of the argument is my own, but I have used Kelly for clarification when I needed him.) According to Kelly 'a person's processes are channelised by the ways in which they anticipate events'. He goes on to say that 'to the extent that one person construes the construction processes of another, they may play a role in a social process involving another person'(1955: 95). The idea is basic to human reality, even if its expression may be a little unfamiliar. Indeed it is more real than some kinds of human experience, because it is fundamental to the creation of the most vital kind of human *personal* reality, that of social relationships between people. In order to be fully human we must possess the ability to experience reality in and through others. At the same time, it is not a basic datum of experience, part of the prime materia of life, because it is essentially an artifact, something put together as a personal approximation of the 'truth' – what Kelly describes as 'personal construct'. To this extent it is a work of conscious art. Just as Goffman regards society as dramaturgically constructed, an artistic attempt at social communication carried on by means of the self-conscious 'presentation' of selected aspects of an over-all inter-personal reality (1971), so Kelly describes a similar process occurring at a micro-social level in which individuals try on for size various views of themselves as perceived by other people, in order to select the ones which allow them to carry on social relationships with one another. Kelly sees our personal role as continually changing as we adjust and readjust our own personal picture of the relationship we want to establish or maintain, in accordance with the principle which 'starts with loosened construction and terminates with tightened and validated construction' (1955: 528). This process of validation involves not simply the provision of an environment which is emotionally secure but one which is structurally recognizable, in which role relationships are clearly defined and different kinds of human experience, laughter, sadness, work, play, formality and informality, are taken in context, each, and each combination of each, receiving validation from recognizable authorities in circumstances widely regarded as being appropriate.

It is here that the artistic nature of social life is seen to be most important. Society can be seen as the conscious and intentional manipulation of personal experience to convey a message about itself. Drama is the image of social process, conveying a message about life in terms of the order it gives to events, mirroring and establishing change. As Goffman pointed out, in daily life the processes whereby this shaping of events is carried out are frequently overlooked or actually hidden from view (1971). In drama these same stratagems of human role playing are clearly revealed; the way life achieves meaning may be studied *in situ*. To this extent drama is both a playground for the release of inter-personal tension and a laboratory for the safe anticipation of events. Even more importantly it provides the clarification of the structures which communicate our experience of social living.

As such it is very relevant to the study of mental illness. The way that some people categorised as schizophrenics think, talk, and relate to other people suggests very strongly that they have difficulty in sharing experiences, and consequently *meanings*, through 'imagining themselves' into someone else's shoes. Such people appear to be suffering from a kind of 'person blindness' according to which they have difficulty in seeing others as at once separate from, and united to, themselves. What Stanislavski characterizes as the 'as if' faculty in human perception seems curiously lacking (1936: 43–49). There is an inability to see the other, without homogenisation or alienation, as *someone else who might be me*. The significance of drama lies in the fact that a person who finds difficulty in giving structure to the way he or she perceives, and consequently thinks, will certainly find the shift from 'it is' to 'it is *as if*' hard to achieve. If I am unable to say 'this is different from that, yet both are significant or meaningful from different points of view or with reference to different criteria of truthfulness', I am unable to move freely among alternative ways of interpreting the world that confronts and contains me. I am unable to make use of one viewpoint as a way of explaining, or expanding, another, and my 'epistemological repertoire' is too limited, and consequently too inflexible for the kind of cross-referencing other people take for granted. This seems to be true of depression as well as of schizoid states.

In both depression and schizophrenia, there is a lack of distance in the experience of people; reality tends to be unitary in the sense of being limited to the here and now, situations are characterized by an overall flatness and two-dimensionality. Drama permits the crucial division between analogy and homology, metaphor and statement to be lived through instead of ignored or circumvented. It does the same thing with the boundary line between people, underlining its presence in order to remove any confusion which might exist between self and other which would render communication otiose.

Drama consists in acting as if I were someone else and knowing that I am doing so. For this reason it is particularly relevant to the kind of thought disorder associated with the schizoid awareness. At the same time it depends on an exchange of personal involvement which depressed people find reassuring. Both the way I perceive the world and the person I am are validated in the interchange of self and other.

This experience is precisely the aim of drama therapy. Just as people leave a theatre in a frame of mind which is eager to embrace the world outside, to engage ideas, situations and people with renewed vigour because of the interpersonal happening in which they have been involved, so people taking part in a drama therapy session are given something to take away in the form of an experience of meaningful human contact. I use the rather vague term quite specifically. The meaning depends on the structure of what happens in the session. Drama therapy, like drama itself, is an arrangement of forms – roles, conventions, contrasts, similarities, modes of understanding, ideas and feelings – which encourages us to discriminate between and choose among a range of different kinds of perception or ways of perceiving.

The argument of this book is that the clearly recognizable structure of drama provides an element of shape which counters existential confusion, confusion about personal identity. That participation in drama has a healing effect has always been recognized.

The implications of this ancient understanding are beginning to be appreciated nowadays more widely than they have been for centuries. In particular, the investigation into drama as healing is being directed in new ways, as our understanding of the dynamics of personal relationship grows. In its ability to handle freedom and structure in ways which allow us to relate to other people without capitulation or denial, drama therapy is able to help all who have difficulty with the phenomenon of inter-personal distance, depressed people who feel themselves threatened and judged by the demands of a more powerful presence than their own, and those schizoid souls who find difficulty in acknowledging any kind of presence really distinct from their own. Drama therapy's contribution lies in its ability to make meaningful distinctions in our awareness of people and to explore the ways in which our personal universes may fit together to provide experiences of personal wholeness. It is a meeting place of selves in a world where such opportunities for communion are scarce – scarcer for some than for others. But this has always been the unique contribution of drama to life. Here are the main points in my argument:

In Chapter One, (Drama as Involvement) the work of Rollo May and other writers who have concerned themselves with the psychology of artistic experience is cited as evidence that drama may be seen as a 'special case' of human relationship, using aesthetic distance as a way of intensifying the mutual involvement of persons. A different point of view is put forward from that of educational drama, which sees drama as an illustrative metaphor for living rather than the substance of life itself, an inevitable part of being human. Drama and theatre depend upon separation of persons – aesthetic distance – which increases psychological interdependence. Because this is so, naturalistic imitation of life is less powerful in its ability to impress than drama distanced by metaphor, whether or not this is embodied in actual physical separation, as it is in theatre. Theatre makes use of our ability to put ourselves in another person's place and 'see' through his or her eyes – an idea first developed by Aristotle in his teaching about *katharsis*, an experience which is able to overcome our isolation and give our ideas the authority of a corporate statement. By demonstrating an alternative reality to our own, drama allows us to revise the way we look at life. This is something on which our psychological health depends, which we often find very difficult.

Chapter Two explores our use of symbols as a mode of inter-personal communication which both protects and extends the self. Object Relations Theory supports the claim that human awareness develops according to a growing ability to 'handle' distance. The idea of theatre as a space *between*, an area of experiment between 'me' and 'not me', introduced in Chapter One, is further developed, this time from a psychological point of view. Winnicott's notion of the 'transitional object' links ideas of play, safety, and adventure taking place within a specially structured framework and leading to the growth of relationship with other people. Even in later life such 'transitional areas' ease relationship (and give rise to a sense of belonging together). Examples apart from theatre are games, adventures into the imagination including 'mystic journeys', or works of literature which draw on ideas of a psychologically 'resonant' kind. Personal Construct Psychology throws light on the part played by the imagination in 'trying the world out for size'. From Kelly's point of view every mental construct is a kind of transitional object, and we are always experimenting, never reaching a final conclusion. We do not do this in isolation, for we construe one another's constructs in an attempt to predict events. Thus we find out about one another as we play one another's games.

Chapter Three begins with a Construct Theory view of depression – depression seen as a lack of psychological flexibility, as a result of which negative judgements about the self are clung onto and positive ones ignored. This may be the result of mothering that was not 'good enough' or of a sense of being unacceptable which has arisen during childhood. Suppressed anger may go back to the Freudian 'oral' stage. This is particularly noticeable in the experience of theatre, where 'under-distanced' individuals find the courage to reveal themselves to other people and the world, and achieve the involvement which will set them free from self-protectiveness. Body experience is particularly important in all this as it is in depression itself.

Chapter Four deals with drama therapy and schizophrenia. Schizophrenics are lacking in ability to see things from a point of view other than their own. In other words, they confuse others with themselves, so that they find it hard to conceive of a network of social relationships among individuals. Bateson and others have claimed that this is due to their having been systematically confused by self-contradictory messages from their parents and so stopped looking for meaning outside themselves. 'Double-bind' situations, 'skewed families', 'processes of mystification', all suggest the systematic breakdown of an individual, personal way of making sense of the world. The link between one's personal view and that of other people has been lost. In accordance with Construct Theory, this means that one's own way of predicting events, always depending on other people's validation, has been seriously damaged, giving rise to the thought disorder which is frequently associated with schizophrenia. This may be modifiable, or even reversible, by a process of systematic validation of constructs within an environment which is safe and reliable and above all, clearly defined, the idea being that a dependable world gives rise to thinking of a consistent kind. Drama therapy aims at producing a reality, or set of realities, which is complex but clearly distinguishable, interesting enough to 'draw us into the action' of validating one another's experiences of the life of relationship. It is particularly relevant to schizophrenia.

Chapter Five opens Part II and concerns important elements within drama therapy. First of all, the combination of structure and freedom, and the importance of scene-setting; secondly, roles, their clarity and flexibility, role-reversal; thirdly, playing games to warm-up, quieten down, break barriers, set limits — a more important activity than might at first be thought; sculpting, using the entire body to express and demonstrate thoughts, feelings, ideas, perceptions; using metaphor or rather, getting used to it, because it is the basic language of art and essential for drama therapy; fitting the process to the individual needs of clients, grading sessions according to the degree of challenge they present (some examples of this are given).

Chapter Six concerns some of the men and women concerned in the drama therapy described and their reactions to it, and Chapter Seven describes sessions themselves, from the point of view of 'observer participation'. It explains why this approach was chosen.

Chapter Eight looks at the connection between drama therapy and ritual, to which it owes much of its healing power, and without which it cannot really be understood. Drama itself has unavoidable religious implications, as Peter Brook and Antonin Artaud have made clear to us. The classical theatres of Greece, India, Japan and the theatrical traditions of many other 'cultures' demonstrate the relationship of drama to religion experienced as healing. Both ritual and drama therapy bring about personal transformation by imaginative means revolving round the use of narrative. Throughout the world religion employs the order of events within the rite to involve men and women in an experience of existential change, often using an actual physical journey to do this. Dramatic ritual is a fundamental religious sign-language, communicating truths unknowable by any other means. Thus, drama therapy puts us in touch with truths lost to a secular age. To do so it needs both theatre and ritual, the first for reformation (re-formation), the second, transformation; it fulfils the function of a transitional object leading those involved into a relationship of ever increasing closeness. Theatre and ritual combine to reverse thinking which is too 'loose' or too 'tight', setting the scene for the willing demolition of barriers against encounter. Currently, there is a movement of renewal in drama therapy; its practitioners are aware of the degree of commitment needed to do justice to so imaginative an approach to psychotherapy.

Drama therapy needs an understanding of both the play and the rite, and of the relationship between them. Embodied imagination about the meaning of life and death, it cannot afford to ignore its identity as part of mankind's personal search for spiritual wholeness.

Part I

Roots

Chapter 1

Drama as Involvement

Insofar as our ordinary, everyday efforts are directed towards making sense of the relationship between self and world, they are creative. Indeed, Rollo May maintains that the creative process itself is in fact a passion for clarity: 'it is the struggle against disintegration, the struggle to bring into existence new kinds of being that give harmony and integration' (1975: 140); that stand out clearly as themselves, and in so doing draw attention to whatever surrounds them so that we see everything more clearly, artifact and setting, figure and ground. To assert the presence of form must be to establish a division, the old division between 'this' and 'that' asserted publicly, demonstrated without confusion. In this way, art creates the space for recognition that leads to understanding. We stand back and look, always metaphorically, sometimes also literally, so that we may perceive everything that is 'there' in the artifact, seeing it as a source of meaning in itself rather than simply part of a well-known perceptual argument. This is the operation that Winnicott refers to as 'creative apperception'. It is this, he says, 'more than anything else, that makes the individual feel that life is worth living' (1971: 65). Far from being an escape from or an evasion of reality, art demands greater engagement with the world. It is produced by men and women as the inevitable expression of their humanity, corresponding to that fundamentally important part of life that sets itself apart to comment on itself. The self about which it wishes to draw conclusions is changed in the process, being given a new identity which can be distinguished from the raw material that went into its construction. This new identity is quite distinct from the old one, although the two exist together, each commenting upon the other and drawing attention to the *difference and similarity* between them. Both realities remain within our experience of life, but the enterprise of re-structuring their relationship brings with it an experience of widened boundaries. Thus a work of art challenges existing structures by its effort to engage human reality at a profounder level of perceptual clarity, that is, of meaning.

This is a very difficult thing to describe, because the process is essentially paradoxical. We distance ourselves (or art distances itself) in order to be engaged with, and involved in, the thing we are standing back from. Rollo May describes it as a way of becoming aware of the essence of an object and revealing it to others: 'Cezanne sees a tree... He experiences, as he no doubt would have said 'being grasped by the tree'. The arching grandeur of the tree, the mothering spread, the delicate balance as the tree grips the earth – all these and many more characteristics of the tree are absorbed into his perception and are felt throughout his nervous structure... This vision involves an omission of some aspects of the scene and a greater emphasis on other aspects and the ensuing re-arrangement of the whole; but it is more than the sum of all these. Primarily it is a vision that is not now tree, but Tree; the concrete tree Cezanne looked at is formed into the essence of tree. However original and unrepeatable his vision is, it is still a vision of all trees triggered by his encounter with this particular one' (1975: 77, 78). The way to an universalised perception of all trees is via an intensified way of perceiving one tree; and the artistic process which opens up a similar experience within the spectator is one of *definition and intensification*.

In a similar way, the kinds of art in which we use our own physical presence as our medium for realising ideas and feelings – drama and theatre – depend upon a high degree of concentration upon their subject matter. An actor 'loses himself' in his part by performing a very definite and precise mental operation of dissociation and association, a shift in his frame of reference corresponding to the temporary adoption of a new 'core role'. In order to 'lose' oneself in this way one must be very sure about what one is losing oneself in; a picture is built up of a new interpretation of a new world, and the business begins of giving that world reality. The process of 'developing a character' is identical with that of elaborating a new way of interpreting reality. The more elaborate the system built up, the more real the portrayal, both for actor and audience. An analogy with the ways in which relationships are formed springs to mind. To form a new relationship is to leap the gap which separates us from someone else; one does not leap unless one is reasonably sure where one will land, even though it never turns out to be exactly the place one had in mind.

The principle is clearly demonstrated in theatre. Here the alternative mental world into which the author invites us is given visible form in the arrangements which distinguish audience from actors – the use of costumes, make-up, masks; stage-settings (particularly if these are non-representational); lighting and sound-effects; above all, the actual physical separation of audience and cast. All these things are real, but the argument which they support is one organised on lines other than the one which governs our customary interpretation of reality. They are here to give structure to the world articulated by the plot, to define it as an artifact, but one fit for human habitation. By demonstrating its own structural difference from the ordinary world, theatre dislodges us from our prepared positions so that we can enjoy the imaginative experience of mutuality and sharing, the expansion of our own private world, which we find so liberating once the barriers are down.[1] The audience is at one and the same time protected and exposed – protected by the fictional, or metaphorical, structure of the event, exposed by the hypnotic fascination of the theatrical image which is focused and intensified by the very things which seem to set it apart from life and render it harmless. The artistic nature of the happening distinguishes two separate but mutually inclusive worlds, brought into relationship by a line of demarcation which unites what it divides, making sense of both. From a technical point of view, theatre may be seen as a way of arranging people and objects to produce the maximum degree of concentration of the human senses. The theatrical 'illusion' has been described as 'the process of confining attention to those involved in a specific situation, of limiting activities…to what is appropriate, or meaningful, or consequential, and observing a defined level of reality. The process is essentially that of providing a frame for action' (Burns, 1972: 17). This is the social reality established by the corporate decision to focus attention on a single set of facts, i.e. those proposed by the action of the play – a process of selection which as Burns points out, is 'inherent in all social action'. It is typified in theatre, where the power of focused humanity creates a kind of reality which takes precedence over other kinds of social awareness. The result is not distortion but the clarification of a particular kind of human awareness, the quality of awareness that makes things real in a personal way.

Theatre is not any kind of imitation of life, but a focused encounter with the personal process involved in living. Its dramatic action is not a metaphor for life, but the way that life works. It can be used metaphorically, as one human situation is used to 'stand for' others with the same underlying significance. This is the way drama teachers are used to regarding it. However, it owes its force to the fact that our behaviour responds particularly well to this sort of interpretation, being intended for it from the beginning.[2] Theatre simply serves to intensify its effects.

The theatre itself, the actual theatre building, is a machine very like a camera; in other words it is a device for achieving the clearest available perceptual image. In the theatre, however, the image is not only visual, but aural as well. In fact it is even more ambitious than this, for it aims at engaging all the senses by using as its medium not light-sensitive film, but the living flesh of human beings. It is here, in the embodied personal event, that healing takes place. In the theatre, the human subject perceives her or his fellow men and women not merely as a two dimensional image printed on a light sensitive plate, but is involved with the object of perception in a unique way, a way that no other 'image intensifier' can hope to emulate. So much is obvious: people and things usually appear more real to us when they are actually present than when we are merely looking at a picture of them.

What is not so obvious, however, is that the theatre manages our perception of the play's characters and plot by actually setting us at a distance from it. The effect of this is to make our involvement all the greater. Several things contribute to this process of setting apart, or differentiating between, 'us' and 'them', the people in the play and those in the audience. To begin with there is the basic difference between two kinds of reality, the ordinary reality of the audience and the extraordinary one of the play, a metaphorical kind of truthfulness, truth expressed in fiction as opposed to literal fact; another place, another time set against the here and now. Secondly, there is the equally important contrast between the way in which what is happening on stage is 'all of a piece', possessing an identifiable beginning and working towards an inevitable conclusion, and the shapelessness of life as we ourselves are conscious of actually being in the process of experiencing it. Life is full of difficulties and confusions, beset by situations which are vague and ill-defined, haunted by the ghosts of dead relationships, preoccupied with our involvement in becoming. The play's structure, its nature as a work of art, comes between us and our ordinary experience, speaking in a language that we recognise about a perfection of meaning to which we aspire. In this way the play directs us to a reality which is both ours and not ours, affording a vision of a truth which we reach out to but are not able to grasp.

It is in the reaching out that healing lies. Certainly the new world of the play is not ours except in imagination. It is the action of sharing it with others that makes it real for us. Reaching out towards the situation which is not our own, but in which we participate, we encounter one another. The difference between the two realities actually encourages this meeting because it draws us out of ourselves towards the other person presented before us in the play. It seems that our imagination thrives on difficulties of this kind, for the play provides us with both a challenge to and a rallying point for an intensified experience of identification. The important thing for us to recognise is the part played in all this by the physical circumstances of the encounter, the theatrical setting itself. Instead of denying these differences, or attempting to cover them up, the staging of plays exploits them. It does this by making use of consciously contrived 'aesthetic distance'[3] in order to secure a richer personal involvement – an involvement which is authentically imaginative *because it cannot be anything else.* It cannot be a literal statement of identity with regard to persons, places or situations in life, for it depends on sympathy with people rather than the simple transmission of ideas taking place on the same level of understanding, as in an ordinary conversation or at a formal lecture or seminar. Thus, as we say, the mechanism which the theatre uses to convey information functions in a way which is multi-dimensional and dialectical. It is an imaginative paradox which unites persons by separating them.

Speaking of the Ancient Greek stage, Martin Buber says that 'we stand inextricably within the event and detached outside it', for theatre is experienced 'not as cleavage or contradiction, but as the polar unity of feelings'. By using formal techniques to exaggerate the distance between two worlds – the world of the play itself, which is literally false but emotionally and imaginatively true, and the everyday literal reality of the audience – the ancient theatre transcended that distance and allowed ordinary people to participate in the poetic truth enshrined in the fictional experiences of its protagonists. The modern theatre uses similar means to obtain the same result. Whatever may be the arrangement of auditorium and acting area the theatre itself, the fact that it *is* a theatre, focuses attention upon the juxtaposition of actors and audience which transforms ordinary attention into involvement.

In Wilshire's words, 'Knowledge of the principles of theatre throws light upon analogous conditions of being human that must be understood before anything else about being a self can be...together actor and audience reconstruct the prototypical organism of human relationship' (1982: 4,24). To study the way that drama and theatre work is to pay attention to the most profoundly important truths about human relationship. Ever since G. H. Mead, psychologists have recognised the vital importance to the individual's own self-interpretation of the thoughts and feelings of other people and particularly of their attitudes towards *him*. The sense of self, Kelly reminds us, is the reflexive awareness which we receive from other people. This goes much further than the mere ability to imagine what other people may be experiencing so that this can be taken into account in organising one's own perceptions: we need to know how they make their own sense, so that we can decide how we will make ours in relationship to them.[4] As Wilshire says, 'one's sense of his own self and mind is derived from his sense of the other's self and mind' (1982: 35). If this is the case, it makes nonsense of the common view of reality which limits it to whatever is observable from a third-person point of view; that is, to entities and events which are objectifiable and can be measured. If we are beings whose personal worlds overlap to this extent, how can we achieve any authentically human view of human matters without distorting the reality we are trying to observe? After all, we *are* the involvement that we wish to discount...

In theatre we are able to examine involvement in an appropriate way, that is, in its own terms, without pretending to ignore it or deceiving ourselves into thinking that we are not subject to its 'distorted' influences. Theatre and drama bring their own clarity to a condition which is too pervasive to be distinguished in any other way. As Wilshire says, 'theatre is an experimental procedure for uncovering mimetic fusion' (1982: 97). It 'speaks the same language' as life, using a fictional scenario of involvement as a key to unlocking a human reality which is itself inescapably transpersonal, and cannot really be understood in any other way. The aim of drama is to put us in touch with the essence of what *really happens* in life, and it is able to do this because what happens in life is dramatic, an imaginative sharing of personal reality.[5]

However the clarity of the perceptual image does not depend on involvement, 'mimetic fusion', alone. It is the human presence of the actors *plus* the mixture of safety and danger, protection and exposure, that we call 'aesthetic distance' that makes the 'as if' real to us. No-one can see clearly if they are so much involved that they do not know what they are doing, although we must know what it is to be involved, to the extent of temporarily losing our sense of independent existence, if we are to recognise it for what it really is. The artificial nature of drama is both defensive and aggressive, drawing us into the action of the drama through its ability to intensify the power of the natural urge to become involved with our own kind, and protecting us from its disturbing force by underlining its identity as fiction. Both these movements contribute to the creative force of theatre, its ability to expand the horizons of our awareness as we struggle with existing limits and seek to define the nature of our experience which occurs spontaneously.

'Creativity', says Rollo May, 'arises out of the tension between spontaneity and limitations' (1975: 115). The same is true of human relationship. The feelings aroused in drama demonstrate the existential anthropology of Martin Buber, according to which the relation 'I – Thou', expressive of involvement, perpetually becomes 'I – It', according to the nature of human consciousness, which withdraws and observes until once more it enters into relation: 'the 'it' is the eternal chrysalis, the 'Thou' the eternal butterfly' (1958: 17). The two movements are mutually dependent: just as 'I – It' depends for its life upon 'I – Thou', so 'I – Thou' requires 'I – It'. The meeting of persons demands the structure of things. Because it never allows us to forget this essential fact, art is the best way for us to look at life. In art, form and content, the known and the unknown, what belongs to the self and what belongs to the other, are experienced in a perceptual oscillation which is not an idea but an event, one which enshrines the living truth of meeting and mutuality. Art communicates the emotion which belongs to the sharing of separate selves, who live in art as they do in life – that is, according to an alternation of 'I – It' and 'I – Thou', a perpetually resolved and reasserted dissonance-and-consonance (1957: 68).

None of this is scientifically demonstrable. All the same, it belongs to common experience. It is a 'fact of life' that we find ourselves in this two-fold experience of yearning for union with others while longing to assert our own individuality. What is claimed here is that theatre acts as a paradigm of this awareness, a natural expression of the terms in which we 'see life', which really means the way we are: 'In witnessing the conditions necessary for persons making sense of the world we (are) witnessing the conditions necessary for persons' existence' (Wilshire, p. 123). Wilshire goes on to say that human meaning requires both fusion with an authoritative source and individuation of one's own experience *as* one's own unique interpretation of life. The first supplies the material for the second. Writing from a totally different standpoint, that of clinical psychology rather than aesthetics, Kelly claims that a person's core role is constructed from the ideas and attitudes of other people, but is nonetheless appropriated as strictly personal, the very essence of self-hood. He uses self-assessment techniques to substantiate his claim. (Kelly 1955: 200ff)[6]

The experience of engulfment by, or fusion in, another person or people – a strictly non-thetic experience – is as necessary to our relationship with the world as is individuation, the 'personal view' which expresses our ability to stand back and draw conclusions. We need to be perpetually united with a source of being recognised as authoritative in order to have the confidence in ourselves to *be* ourselves. Again, this is not immediately demonstrable, but it makes sense of many ordinary experiences of life, as well as confirming what we know about the therapeutic relationship.

It makes striking sense, above all, of drama, and of the imaginative participation in the being of other people which is the primary dramatic phenomenon. Theatre is both challenging and reassuring because it draws on a fundamental mimetic tendency shared by everyone. This is what makes it so appealing to us, so that we find ourselves taking part in the dramatic action even against our will, swept up in whatever is happening before us. The effect of drama, as Aristotle pointed out, is an emotional purging or katharsis. In other words, our way of perceiving the world is purified by the intensity of our emotional involvement in the play. He regarded the theatre as a kind of safety valve: it restores our emotional balance by bringing certain feelings to the surface and giving them the expression that they demand, and which is usually denied them. Specifically, the two emotions mentioned by Aristotle are pity and fear: 'Pity and fear, artificially stirred, expel the latent pity and fear which we bring with us from real life, or at least such elements in them are as disquieting, (for) the regulated indulgence of the feelings serves to maintain the balance of nature' (1894: 254).

There is still life in the ancient formula. Aristotle does not claim that pity and fear are somehow expelled or got rid of by the theatre, but that they are purified and refined by it, so that they become health-inducing emotions instead of debilitating or destructive ones. In the *Rhetoric* he defines fear as 'a species of pain or disturbance arising from an impression of impending evil which is destructive or painful in its nature; the evil is near and not remote, and the persons threatened are ourselves.' Similarly, pity is 'a sort of pain at an evident evil of a destructive or painful kind in the case of someone who does not deserve it; the evil being one which we might expect to happen to ourselves, or to some of our friends, and this at a time when it is seen to be near at hand.'[7]

'One which we might expect to happen to ourselves'. The effect of involvement in the imaginative world of the theatre is to modify the nature of the emotions caused by events which happen in the real world. Instead of being turned inwards upon the self, painful feelings are projected outwards onto the characters of the play. The important thing to realise, however, is that even though they are projected outwards, these feelings of distress are not simply denied or disowned, because of the sympathetic involvement which takes place with the stage characters, who are like ourselves but not ourselves. Beholding them and the situation in which they are placed, the nature of our fear is transformed by our pity; that is, our fear for ourselves is no longer simply the natural apprehension and anxiety we feel about our own life, revealed in all its vulnerability and precarious frailty by the action taking place before us, it is also the sympathy we cannot help feeling for others like us, in the same position as us.

Thus theatre's healing effect is in its relational nature. His description of the emotional effect of theatre upon the spectator seems to suggest a kind of 'universalization of the emotions', an experience of human solidarity with other people as a whole, not simply the individual actor with whom we empathise. Seen like this, theatre is a way of gaining the courage to exist alongside one's fellow women and men, because it is able to liberate both the actor and the spectator from a crippling pre-occupation with self, so that we are enabled to see ourselves in our proper context as people who draw strength from one another because, at the most essential level of all, we belong together.

Those whose job it is to try and ease the pain of people who have emotional problems and the psychological burdens associated with them are well aware of this effect of theatre. There are many ways in which theatre can be used to produce a healing katharsis, some of which do not even involve the use of a real stage and living actors. The one described here is only intended as an example of a range of techniques:

> Those taking part cut pictures of various 'characters' from illustrated magazines, and arrange them on the stage of a toy theatre, set on a table at one end of the room. People are encouraged to put the characters on the stage in no particular order, and to invent a story line which will explain their relationship to one another and their reason for appearing in the scene. A period of *ad hoc* experimentation follows when the figures are moved around on the stage in order to try to produce the kind of relationship between characters out of which a plot may be contrived. Soon, the interest of the group quickens as people start acting out the story they themselves have created for themselves, using the space in front of the toy theatre as an improvised acting area. The play that eventually emerges is a kind of synthetic creation, in which the fictional story that has been contrived from the toy theatre and its magazine characters is transformed by the force of the actors' own personal experience, and

personal biography is subjected to the power of imaginative identification with the situations of others.

It is on these terms that drama comes alive. A vital transaction takes place of an Aristotelian kind. The actors involved both receive life from the play and give life to it, endowing the fictional characters with their joy and suffering. Individuals emerge refreshed, having for however short a time lost themselves in finding somebody else. This simple experimental game reveals something vital about the nature of theatre. A fictional story universalizes an emotion which is deeply private, intensely personal, as the natural pity which we feel for someone else with whom we are emotionally involved loosens the grip of self and releases us, albeit temporarily, from our preoccupation with our own pain.[8]

The kind of pain from which we find release in drama is the insecurity and vulnerability of our existential isolation. Psychologically speaking, it allows us to measure our private ways of making sense of life with what is going on in the play and to take comfort from the recognition of the common ground that exists, in the way of thoughts and feelings of actual events. Kelly speaks of life experiences which have the effect of confirming us in the ability to make sense of the world, on which our sense of ourselves depends. (1955: 157ff). To use Wilshire's term, in our involvement with others we seek *authorisation*, 'permission to be' (1982: 6, 7). The lives of the characters in the play are part of the shared experience of mankind, structured to give them the clarity and definition which both sets them apart from us and draws us in to the meaning and purpose that they embody.

The intentionality of art, its concern to make some kind of definitive statement about human reality, has the effect of making drama a powerful source of authorisation for those involved, who, as human beings, naturally interpret life in terms of learning *from* and learning *about*, fusion and individuation. We confirm one another in selfhood by a process of imaginative involvement in one another's experience, making that experience partly our own, and in so doing authorising the other person in possession of it. Upon this reflexive process of giving and receiving depends our ability to live in relationship with other people, and, consequently, our ability to make sense of life.[9] If we find it difficult to achieve, we need help in achieving it.

This is the level at which drama and theatre are most 'true' and consequently most valuable as therapy. It is born out by the testimony of people who study drama from several angles – the sociological, psychological and aesthetic as well as the theatrical. As a source of authorisation and individuation art reveals its real significance, not as any kind of *imitation* of life but as *participation* in the essential processes of human experience. The use of drama as a therapeutic medium makes the relationship between self and other, 'I-for-myself' and 'I-from-others' explicit, for I can establish myself *as* myself, as separate from others who participate in my self-awareness, simply by acting them. By acting other people I establish myself as a person with regard to them, and consequently as a person for myself. My words and gestures constitute the triumph of individuality over engulf-ment, and by using an obvious contrivance, a situation which has been deliberately structured, I am able to distinguish some of the principles which determine my characteristic way of reacting to other people, the terms of my involvement in what Laing, Phillipson and Lee have called the 'spiral of perspectives' which holds me so tightly in its grip (1966).

The most important thing of all about drama is that it allows us to revise the way in which we look at life. It does this by demonstrating the contingent nature of our attitudes and arrangements, the 'view of life' which we use in order to predict events. 'To stage a drama,' says Wilshire, 'is to intervene in the circuit of life and to build a model of it which disturbs life even as we find it conforming to the model... The play demonstrates how we cast ourselves, or are cast by others, in life. It is the mission of art to reveal this off-stage reality' (1982: 209). Drama allows us to practice what Kelly calls 'constructive alterna-tivism' – the assumption that all of our present interpretations of the universe are subject to revision or replacement (1955: 15). We can accept or reject new ideas about life in a way and at a level of understanding which passes ordinary argument and brings home the actual reality of the choices to be considered. Whatever we choose to do or to be, we can receive the message about choice in a practical way because it is encoded in a language with which we are deeply familiar, one which we understand and respond to with all of ourselves, and not just the critical intellect.[10] In Construct Theory terms, the techniques which we employ in order to separate different kinds of social reality in the service of a particular definition of a situation represent an ability which to some degree or other we all possess as human beings, that of distinguishing between different parts of our overall view of life ('construct sub-systems'), and according a different kind of reality to each of them. In terms of Kelly's 'Fragmentation Corollary', 'A person may successively employ a variety of construction sub-systems which are inferentially incom-patible with one another' (1955:83f). Drama is, I maintain, a way of validating this ability and of strengthening it in the case of those who find its exercise difficult.

In some cultures the public use of alternative, sometimes contradictory, 'sub-systems of self presentation' is better organised and more socially acceptable than it is in others.[11] The fewer public, official, definitions of social reality there are, the more opportunity there is for private, unofficial ones. There seems no reason to believe that under ordinary circumstances this should cause individual men and women any real trouble, so long as they are able to make reasonably clear decisions about the ways in which they are going to define various social situations, in order to react appropriately to them. Nobody need use all of his or her personal reality at any time; indeed the attempt to 'take too much in' tends to result in shortage of adequate structures for the prediction and control of events and consequent anxiety. Certainly, from a psychological point of view it seems preferable that we should be aware of what we choose to disregard, even when this involves us in holding two contradictory positions at once. Both may contribute in different ways to our total view of 'the truth'. After all, as Kelly maintains, there are not only different levels of importance in construing, but different 'ranges of convenience' for the constructs we use: an interpretation which clarifies one area of experience may distort our view of another. This is not something we *can* do, but something we *must* do in order to survive socially, and therefore personally. Sanity, in fact, may be the ability to believe two mutually contradictory things at the same time. The key would certainly seem to be our ability to recognise the contingent nature of various kinds of reality. In other words, our ability to behave 'as if'.[12]

I have drawn attention to two complementary experiences which belong to the nature of drama, and perhaps of all art. The feelings of satisfaction and serenity which come from a play that 'moves' us have to do with the experience of losing our separate identities in an experience of emotional involvement, a shared experience of common life; while our ability to integrate these feelings and to translate them into ideas that we can use for the future belongs to the movement of withdrawal and detachment in which we recognise the play as an artefact, something contrived, useful and satisfying to the heart and mind, perhaps causing us to reflect a little upon the contingent nature of 'reality', but possessing no final authority except that of a powerful metaphor. Both movements are necessary; without the possibility of withdrawing we would never allow ourselves to get involved and run the risk of forfeiting our independent selfhood. The contrived artistic nature of the play permits us to distance ourselves from ourselves in order to see beyond ourselves and really look at – and feel for – another person. Within the structure of the play we feel both safe and challenged. Drama makes a firm distinction between two kinds of reality, and tells us clearly that neither of them has a final hold over us. Within the limits of a structure which is clearly perceived and understood, it provides a comparatively safe 'middle ground' between private fantasy and public reality, allowing a limited engulfment in other people, and a ready-made identity within an obvious structure. We shall explore this idea in more depth in the next chapter.

Notes

1. The existentialist philosopher Martin Buber describes this phenomenon in his essay on the staging of Greek tragedy, where he suggests that the presence of space between Theatron and Skene contributed powerfully to the identification of actors and audience, producing an effect of 'polar unity' arising out of 'the stern over-againstness of I and Thou' which constitutes relationship (1957: 67, 72). The distancing effect of theatrical presentation, the ways in which it sets about shaping its own separate world, induce a relaxation of the structures which we use to define our own personal reality. 'Aesthetic distance', says Wilshire, 'regulates the intercourse of 'world' and world. It is just because of this protection that the audience can uncover itself at its most vulnerable levels: its archaic mimetic fusions with others' (1982: 23).

2. cf. Burke, 1968: 'Drama is...a fixed form that helps us discover what the implications of the term 'act' and 'person' *really are*' (p 448).

3. This is not to be confused with psychological distance, which simply means separation. Aesthetic distance often implies the action of withdrawing from something or someone in order to study it or them in a cooler, more detached, way. In fact the opposite may happen, as we become more, rather than less, involved, as we concentrate thoughts and feelings away from ourselves. This is particularly so in the theatre, where 'distance' demonstrably 'lends enchantment'. See Landy (1986), Schaff (1980)

4. 'A good deal is accomplished in any therapeutic series when the client develops a more adequate understanding of how the others with whom he lives are viewing their worlds. His enactment of a revised role follows immediately upon this reconstruction' (1955: 1141).

5. Wilshire regards mimesis as fundamental to human awareness, rather than seeing it as an epiphenomenon, 'the product of the transference', as psychoanalysis assumes it to be. Instead, the transference itself is here regarded as a special case of the mimetic instinct. To use theatre as a way of understanding life is an experimental procedure, says Wilshire, because of the 'epistemological parity of 'world' (i.e. the world of the play) 'and world' (1982: 102). He claims very convincingly that theatre or the theatrical approach, provides the means for the only authentically scientific study of human life.

6. Kelly used a technique known as the 'repertory grid' (1955). See Glossary.

7. *Rhetoric*, 2/5/13829/21 & 2/8/13856/13.

8. It should perhaps be noted that the doctrine of katharsis has not always been accepted by scholars and critics of the theatre, who have tended to condemn its dependence on the emotions rather than the intellect. Fontenelle, writing in the 17th Century complains that he himself has 'never been able to understand how the passions are purged by the passions themselves'. On the other hand, Antonin Artaud completely rejected the idea of theatre as the prosaic imitation of ordinary reality: 'Art is not the imitation of life. Life is the imitation of a transcendent principle with which art restores communication.' His idea of theatre was of the powerful presence of an 'irrational and gratuitous life-force' possessing a 'reality of its own, a spatial, sensory double of the intellectual, giving another form to reality.' In Artaud's view, the intellect and the emotions exist side by side, but the truth of the latter is inevitably masked by the former's pretensions to being the source of final truth about life. The tremendous gift bestowed by the theatre lies in its ability to remove the intellectual defences that we erect against the healing force of our emotions. There is, he tells us, a fundamental sense of life which can only be attained when our habitual assumptions about 'reality' have been removed; and the only way to remove them is by a direct frontal attack upon them. The authority which the world of common sense exercises over our imagination must be temporarily removed, by creating an alternative reality which will be, for the time being at least, actually more real, more convincing, than everyday life. The idea of a theatre which in the violence of the events it portrays and the threatening

nature of the ideas it expresses is genuinely 'larger than life' has been shown to have great possibilities in psychotherapy as a kind of psychological exorcism.

9. According to Heidegger, the ability of the self to fall into step with others mimetically and to take over their attitudes towards itself is one of the 'categorical potentialities' of human beings (1962).

10. However, so far as our ability to think critically about the world goes, drama certainly helps us to make sense of the structures of society. According to Harré and Secord 'the model of a man as an actor putting on a performance is not only useful and valuable as a model, but in fact represents what goes on in many life situations' (1972: 315); and Goffman states firmly that: 'life itself is a dramatically enacted thing' (1971: 78). This idea has been extensively used by Goffman, whose 'Dramaturgical Theory of Social Analysis' depends on an examination of the manipulation of theatrical structures in non-theatrical settings for the purpose of defining various kinds of social interaction. We 'build our own stages' in order to present the view of ourselves and our intentions which we want others to accept. Life is not simply mimetic in essence, it is very definitely staged in practice: 'The issues dealt with by stagecraft and stage-management are sometimes trivial, but they are quite general: they seem to occur everywhere in social life, providing a clear-cut dimension for formal sociological analysis' (1971: 26).

11. Harré and Secord draw attention to Japan as an example of a culture in which the situational presentation of self is considerably better organised than it is in western Europe (1972: 143).

12. In fact, role playing would seem to depend on scenarios rather than cultures. Certainly, society may make it easier for people to see their own individuality reflected and confirmed by others by providing an extensive repertoire of different kinds of recognisable roles of an official or semi-official nature. However, many if not most roles are simply invented by the men and women who find themselves playing them. They emerge from the situation itself and owe as much to the basic human ability to structure whatever may happen to one, or to exploit structural elements within a given state of affairs in order to make proper sense of it. There are many different kinds of role, apart from institutional ones within recognised social units; some endure only as long as a single social encounter, some last a lifetime; some are invented, some inherited; most importantly, many are pragmatic combinations of former roles. Many of these structures, although drawn from and reflected by, other people, are kept discreetly apart from them: It doesn't really matter if a person is unaware of the way I see myself with regard to him, the role I have given myself in his particular drama, or indeed the role I have cast *him* in! It is real to me, and may be an essential part of the way I structure my own personal universe.

Chapter 2

The Healing Symbol

In one form or another every human being employs symbols to express things outside the immediate range of their present situation. Whether in the form of verbal metaphor, bodily gesture, or the shape given to a series of actions, symbolism is a way of reaching out from one's association with, or inclusion in, one way of being in order to summon an alternative one, at least in thought and imagination. Thus it links engulfment and individuation, as the action of reaching out is an assertion of independence. The phenomenon of aesthetic distance that we have been considering is a special case of 'psychic distance' which, says Susan Langer 'allows us to apprehend through symbol what was not articulated before.' Symbols arise 'as a consequence of distancing or detaching the self from the object' (1951: 223). In one form or another, they constitute the means whereby we are able to look at life from an individual point of view and draw our own conclusions from it, using our ability to perceive and think about, an objective referent which is contacted via the symbol but does not depend on it. Symbols which are shared nevertheless remain personal.

Langer's view is reminiscent of Object Relations Theory, which sees the symbol as the most important way in which the gap between persons is bridged. The 'object' referred to is 'the thing in regard to which, or through which, the instinct is able to achieve its aim' (Freud, 1915: 122). The first object is the breast, but the development of a child's ability to form a 'mental picture' of his or her mother leads to the first real relationship: 'when symbolism is employed the infant is already clearly distinguishing between fantasy and fact, between inner and external events' (Winnicott, 1971: 6). A symbol is a mental presence which draws attention to an absence and serves in part to make up for it. In other words, symbols participate in that to which they point. They are the link we have with what is not ourself and can never be included 'within' us. Failure to be able to symbolise has been associated with schizophrenia, a condition in which 'the inability to make any links between inner and outer worlds is seen in its full malignancy' (Winnicott, 1976: 222). People in such a position have nothing authentically 'apart' from themselves to compare and contrast things with; they retain an undifferentiated awareness.[1] At every stage in one's life it is necessary to draw upon the security of this original state, the narcissistic omnipotence of the first months, in which everything and everyone that existed was known to be part of oneself. The quality of the nurturance a child receives influences the quality of the basic trust he or she develops.[2] On this original experience of total security, eventual autonomy as a person depends, and consequently the clarity of the boundaries established between the individual and the world, boundaries that define that world for him or her. Much hangs on the individual's success in dealing with the transition from this to a more differentiated existence: indeed it is this transition that makes him or her an individual. With the help of what Winnicott calls 'good-enough mothering', 'it is possible for the individual to cope with the immense shock of loss of omnipotence' involved in the 'transition from a stage of being merged with the mother to a state of being in relation to the mother as something outside and separate' (1971: 71, 15).

Surely this kind of dependence characterises depressed people as well as those who develop in a schizoid way. I cannot find any accounts of this in the literature but it seems most likely that a similar kind of confusion about boundaries plays a part in the life long involvement with the attitudes and opinions of other people which leads depressed people to seek approval so desperately. Certainly the world of the depressed is clearly defined, but that does not make it any more assimilable. Like a schizoid person, a chronic depressive has difficulty in making use of the distinction between self and other on which relationship depends. In this case, however, the boundary seems to be too high – they cannot reach across it and retain their own selfhood. They can certainly get across, but at the cost of leaving themselves behind. Like schizophrenics they have difficulty in holding the two spheres of awareness, self and not-self, in tension, the creative tension that characterises healthy awareness. The depressed person seeks to validate his or her own being by drawing life from the being of others, a life which seems so much more important than their own. They are abnormally concerned with the feelings, attitudes and opinions of those around them, attributing more significance, more *value* to them than they do their own products. Thus the ordinary give-and-take of life is problematic for them, as for schizoid people, and they end up having difficulty doing either. Without the self confidence to assimilate what they receive and make it their own, they feel they have nothing of their own to give – nothing that is worth having, at any rate. This condition is the mirror-image of the schizophrenic one. Instead of losing the other in the self, we lose ourselves in the other. In both cases there is a fundamental boundary confusion.

Here we see the relevance of Object Relations Theory to the argument about the psychological significance of art, for it provides an explanation of the part played by the creative imagination in producing the kind of structurally differentiated personal universe

– what Kelly would call a 'permeable construct system' – on which healthy personal
relationships depend. To facilitate this process, the 'space between' is taken up by an
experience which is neither fusion nor separation, but involves both of these things in
an oscillation of 'me' and 'not me'. This corresponds to an area of transition, intervening
between two kinds of wholeness, that of knowing nothing outside the self, and that of
being in relationship with other selves. Without the proper establishment of the first kind
of identity the emerging self will remain unsure of its individual outline and tend to see
the world as part of itself, to be interpreted and controlled according to its own wishes.
Private fantasy will continue to dominate its mental activity and the ability to think
abstractly – that is away from the self and its immediate sensations – will have difficulty
in developing. Because of the vagueness and lack of definition associated with the
all-important distinction between self and not-self, other boundaries which serve to
define human experience may be vague as well. Having never learned to make this first
vital distinction, it continues to live in an undifferentiated universe – or at least its personal
experience is unlikely to be as clearly differentiated as that of other people who, as a
result of adequate emotional security during the first months of life, have been able to
confront the terrifying awareness of a world 'out there', and so pass across the first real
frontier they have ever encountered. On the other hand, as we have seen, too firm a
distinction may make independent existence equally difficult.

The way in which this process of 'secondary identification' is achieved is considered
to be of the very greatest importance. For the emerging self the gradual erosion of
omnipotence and the loss of invulnerability that goes along with it must necessarily be
a terrifying prospect. Rollo May regards it as something we never really recover from;
having once quit the safety of a totalitarian subjectivity in order to participate in the life
of others we find ourselves in a position 'between the devil and the deep blue sea', terrified
of being totally subsumed by the reality in terms of which we understand our own
independence, and in which we live as persons. The fear of 'life' is counterbalanced by
the fear of 'death': 'all our lives we oscillate between these two fears – *Life* fear is fear of
living autonomously, *death* fear is fear of being totally absorbed by the other' (1975: 19).
Winnicott stresses the need to take account of the paradox inherent in the transition
between total subjectivity and the acceptance of objective reality without attempting to
resolve it. We can neither abide in the experience of fusion nor leave it. Both self and
other must gain reality from the relationship between them. This paradox is fundamental
to human awareness. Its resolution results in my first work of art as an individual – the
Promethean action according to which my uniqueness is asserted and established. This
new creation reflects me and participates in my own inalienable reality, but is not me, as
it demonstrably exists in its own right. In other words, I select an object in the outside
world and bestow an identity upon it, so that, despite being mine, it now 'belongs to

itself',[3] and this first and foremost is achieved by learning to play. Playing is an unique way of being, a reality of its own with a special significance for human affairs. It is not to be confused with other kinds of experience, although it affects the quality of all experience. Winnicott describes it like this: 'This area of playing is not inner psychic reality. It is outside the individual, but it is not in the external world – the child gathers objects or phenomena from external reality and uses them in the service of some sample derived from inner or personal reality' (1971: 51). According to this model, imaginative play is the key both to human relationship and to art. It is an important means of making personal contact with the environment of people and things. It functions as a link between personal realities, for its symbolic nature leads us outward from ourselves into participation in the other and back again to ourselves, our frame of mind subtly changed by the experience. It counters the tendency to concentrate on a private universe or capitulate to the will of others and merely imitate their actions. What begins as an exercise in self-expression, the celebration of one's own abilities, leads into an experience of self-expansion and self-elaboration, as we become aware of the potentialities implicit in our relationship with all that is not ourselves. The movement of fusion and the complementary one of withdrawal belong to the original transition from an undifferentiated awareness of the self to an ability to distinguish, predict and control. We may say that art enables us to share the experience of autonomy and dependence, so that we may lose and find ourselves in ways that seem safe because we ourselves have contrived them. The therapeutic importance suggested by phenomenology is underlined by psychoanalysis.

'Transitional objects' are both defensive and aggressive, as they attempt to control a threatening situation, and this dual purpose persists into later life as a main characteristic of art, which both imposes form on, and draws form from, objects. The beneficial influence of an urge to form which is able to find no satisfactory or adequate expression when it is focused directly upon the artist's emotional life are reflected back upon him – and upon others – by the works of art he produces. The separation of the symbol from both of its referents, subject *and* object, is able to influence our psychic experience, as it were from outside, from an independent reality, or rather one to which we have given independence. The transitional object is a thing, an artefact; we are able to stand back from it as something completely apart from ourselves, possessing no power over us. At the same time we have endowed it with human significance, so that it represents our own humanity, which is open to the seductive humanity of other people. To involve ourselves in it is to fuse our life with theirs, while retaining our own individuality. The distinction within human experience represented by transitional objects is of the very greatest importance, standing as it does for an existential decision of inestimable consequence. All other genuine decisions depend on this one. From now onwards we are committed to a way of being which is both separate from and involved in other people and must learn to organise our perceptions in accordance with the sophisticated systems which human beings find themselves using when they attempt to make sense of one another from a position in which subject and object, examiner and examined, are interchangeable, and I am as much aware of your view of me as I am of my own view of you.

In our own Western culture, transitional objects help us come to terms with the reality of people whom we have permitted to be genuinely other, genuinely independent of ourselves. The price we pay is the terror of being taken over by something we ourselves have created. The reward, however, is an end to isolation and loneliness. If I cannot find the courage to take this step, I may never again find the courage to venture outside my own boundaries. I may have lost the key to whole-hearted participation in life, which lies in the ability to lose the self in the other in order to establish the other in the self. Fatally unsure of myself at this early stage of my life, I may spend all of my life more or less alone.

It is through imaginative games, as G. H. Mead points out, that we develop an awareness of ourselves and our relationship to others. By playing at Mum or Dad we learn that they are significantly different from ourselves and yet importantly similar. When we come to play team games, the process continues, for we are unable to join in without learning to see how our own actions fit into the overall pattern of the two teams, our own and the opposing one. This is certainly a key concept for any consideration of the dramatic relationship, the imaginative game which is both safe and dangerous, familiar and strange, reassuring and challenging – the symbol which separates and unites. Here, in imagination, we experiment with the future and re-live the past without committing ourselves to either. Imagination is not fantasy, because it concerns reality in the form of images and ideas relating directly to past experience and future action. Because the products of the individual imagination in its mediated form as words, images, sounds, textures etc. are available to others, it constitutes a kind of privileged area for the formation of relationships, possible linkages existing in hypothetical circumstances prior to estab- lishment as part of a public reality. Art itself depends on this process, and the 'creative therapies' based on specific art-forms – music, dance, the visual arts and drama – concentrate on the use of imagination to provide the setting for their activities.

The imagination does more than this, however. It leads us beyond the prosaic reality of our conscious awareness into areas of our awareness of life and death, god and mankind which refer to a deeper knowledge, a profounder reality – the sphere of dreams and nightmares. The relationship between dream states and the waking imagination is a shadowy one, but most people are familiar with the experience of having vivid and disturbing dreams after reading a particular book or visiting the cinema to see a horror movie. Evenings at the theatre can provide a dramatic example. Carl Jung directs our attention to a list of stories and plays particularly likely to have a frightening effect because of their ability to activate psychic material which has been specifically denied to consciousness.[4] The terror proceeded, he said from the ability of certain images to relate at an unconscious level to the part of the individual psyche which has become 'split off' or disowned by consciousness while remaining attached to him or her like a shadow. The 'shadow' is the archetype of all intrusive presences and unwelcome reminders; it is the element which by definition has to be kept out of the light of common day. It is only one archetype among many however. The ultimate effect of our making conscious contact with any of these 'dominants of the collective unconscious' is to move us nearer towards psychic integrity. Some archetypes have a comforting or reassuring effect. The shadow is one of those that relates to the so-called 'dark side' of our individual psyches, bringing it a little farther into the light of consciousness and so restoring our psychic balance.[5]

If an archetypal image terrifies us, this is because we have refused to acknowledge the threatening personal reality it awakes in us. Jung tells us that material relating to archetypes enters our awareness by means of our image-making faculty, which he calls the 'imaginatio'. As the 'active evocation of inner images' (1953: 462), imagination is able to give a meaning to chaos, and to present this to us in the form of dreams, visions, fantasies, and every kind of art. 'He who speaks in primordial images...transmutes our personal destiny into the destiny of mankind, thereby evoking in us all those beneficent forces that have always enabled mankind to find a refuge from every peril and to outlive the longest night ...'. That, says Jung, 'is the secret of effective art' (1928: 248).[6]

A powerful image of psychic healing is the one known as the 'mystic journey'. This occurs in one form or another in most cultures. Journeys have obvious therapeutic significance; we wish to move away from our present condition and to enter a sphere of increased wholeness and health. The mystical element represents the heart of the healing process; we journey in to the 'centre' and out again. The archetype here is the journey itself, the symbol of a healing process. Its most dramatic expression is in shamanic religions. The shamanic ecstasies described by Eliade involve 'the leaving of the body and the mystical journey to Heaven or Hell' (1960: 62),[7] in order to bring back power and inspiration for healing. In the imaginative experience of drama therapy groups the journey is an essentially corporate experience. At the same time, the leader of the group plays an essential role as the link between earth, hell and heaven as this is presented in the potent symbolism of the 'journey' (see pp. 86f).

Whether or not the idea of the collective unconscious and its archetypes has meaning for us, the psychological power possessed by symbols of wholeness in works of art, whether this is mediated by a particular image or by the work's overall organisation and interior relationships, has an integrating effect upon us. It is as if we are drawn out of ourselves, towards a larger wholeness, a more perfect harmony. Art expresses a poetic possibility, suggesting much more than it says. The greater the work of art, the more noticeable the sense of something unexpressed. It is by reminding us of the inexpressible that art heals.

The therapeutic use of art has this experience of 'being led out of oneself' as its main aim. Once it has been aroused, our imagination not only shows us different worlds, but encourages us to explore them. We do not necessarily have to do this alone, for the imagination has a contagious quality, so that our own takes wing more swiftly in the presence of that of other people. This happens strikingly in dramatic experience – we shall see that it underlies the therapeutic use of drama – but it is the basis of all the arts, and the therapies associated with them. Whether works of art are transitional objects linking self to other without danger of loss of identity, or potent symbols mediating an awareness of relationship at the deepest level of our being, they remain the principal product of the creative imagination as it sets about its task of making personal sense out of the raw material of our instinctual life.

So far as the psychology of artistic experience goes, no approach has proved more illuminative than George Kelly's Construct Theory (1955). Kelly describes how, with the development of the imaginative faculty that permits us to 'play' our way into relationship, we can begin to organize our own personal view of life, one which will make sense of the relationship between the world and ourselves. It is an artistic process that lasts as long as life itself. 'Each person', says Kelly, 'devises as best he can a structure for making sense of a world of humanity in which he finds himself…he makes social predictions on the basis of this construction…without such patterned structure it would appear that no man can come to grips with his seething world of people, nor can he establish himself as a psychological entity.' Linked to this is the equally vital proposition that '*all of our present interpretations of the universe are subject to revision or replacement*' (1955: 15).

Thus, he brings dramatic experience into the very centre of the study of human psychology, for the world of drama is 'constructive alternativism' incarnate. Construct systems are the *mises en scene* for the drama of human relationship, the cast and setting for a plot that is always changing, always changeable. Observer and observed are mutually involved and reciprocally active, and meaning emerges from the relationship between them rather than being manufactured by one out of material provided by the other. Of all psychologists, Kelly takes this fact most seriously. With his 'credulous approach' to the self-reporting of others, he starts out from a point of view which takes full account of the scientific probity of 'as if'. Each character in the social drama must be understood as being concerned to put forward their own unique point of view in order for the play to have any meaning.

A closer look at Kelly's approach may help us understand the interchange of awareness involved in human relationship. According to him, our understanding of the other person is achieved by the process of construing his or her world. This does not mean merely having an idea or a concept of someone else's way of interpreting life. The notion of a concept, he claims, is far too limiting to be useful as a tool for understanding people, particularly if it is taken to mean 'a construction comprising separate and distinguishable entities which are verbally symbolised.' People put things together to make sense of them long before they can talk, and continue to do so even longer afterwards. The most primitive cognitive act of all, that of distinguishing 'this' from 'that', requires no language at all, and yet it turns out to be the most important thing we ever do in life 'for every experience, to the extent that it stands out at all, stands out in terms of its similarities and distinctions' (1962: 199). This is the basic psychological construct. At a higher level of perceptual organisation, we make sense of the world according to the properties or attributes we assign to, or recognise in, things, people and events. We understand reality in terms of a network of contrasts which provides us with a range of pathways for action in the world, as in every situation which confronts us we decide which is the 'preferred role' (i.e. 'this' as distinct from 'that') of the construct involved, and organise our perceptions on that basis.

Seen like this, human beings are always experimenting, to the extent that they are ceaselessly involved in testing hypotheses in the attempt to make sense of the world. 'A person's processes are psychologically channelized by the ways in which he anticipates events' (1955: 103). This sense is experienced as available in the world, not imposed upon it.[8] At every level of experience we are engaged in following a maze through life, as we systematically choose between alternatives which lie before us. Even the resolution to do nothing, or to compromise, involves us in choice. We predict what will happen if we choose one way, and if our prediction is validated by events, the grounds upon which we made it are strengthened, and this part of our construct system is rendered more stable as a consequence. On the other hand, an invalidated construct is weakened and we look round for another way of construing what has happened to us. At such times we may fall back on a more important construct: more important, that is, with regard to its function within the total interpretative system which we use with regard to ourselves, other people and the world in general. If our experience of construct invalidation has not affected this 'core construct' – has not weakened our confidence that our customary way of making sense of life is a valid one – then we may rest in this knowledge while we re-interpret the situation which baffles us in other ways, using other constructs.

A construct is essentially something that need not necessarily be applicable to the reality it is being used to make sense of. When we construe we use hypotheses which we temporarily *assume to be* true, and make specific predictions from them; but if these do not materialise we are usually free to abandon that construct as inappropriate for the occasion and look elsewhere for a more suitable interpretation. A construct is, after all, only a tool, to be taken up when it seems likely to be useful and laid aside again when no longer needed. Most constructs are useful sometimes (although the scope of any one of them may be limited to the interpretation of a particular kind of event). However if they are constantly invalidated – if the event they are used to predict rarely happens – they begin to lose their credibility.

Thus the whole system is flexible, change at one level affecting the overall organisation, as the system adapts to meet new circumstances and make sense of what is going on at present and seems most likely to happen in the future. In practical terms, the purpose of the whole enterprise is one of *prediction*; by tying in the present with the past in this way we gain some kind of purchase upon the future. By having flexible connections within a stable framework of likely events we are prepared for eventualities while remaining capable of adapting to surprises – that is, to situations we had not expected, and which would otherwise confound us.

Kelly describes the variations in the way in which construct systems function in terms of the strength or weakness of their inner connections – that is the relationships between constructs and their ability to affect one another in order to make the whole system more, or less, efficient as a predictor of events. 'Loose' systems, in which constructs are only vaguely associated, change easily but tend towards instability, so that the person concerned has difficulty in drawing firm conclusions from them. (We shall return to this idea later, when we are considering schizoid states.) 'Tight' systems are much more rigorously organised, so that the slightest connections between constructs are an integral part of the system which tends to change less easily and to be 'all of a piece', each construct being interpreted in terms of the whole network of relationships. In Kelly's terms such systems 'lead to unvarying predictions' (1955: 483) simply because everything is understood as providing evidence for a single overriding proposition about the nature of the universe. In people who are psychologically normal this kind of certainty belongs to the core structures only; nothing is likely to shake their deepest convictions and firmest habits, but other parts of the system are open to modification in ways that do not affect the integrity of the whole.

Notes

1. Eric Fromm describes the normal process of identification through which it is supposed that this separation is achieved: 'Slowly the child comes to regard the mother and other objects as entities apart from itself. Through its own activity (it) experiences a world outside itself' (1960: 20).
2. E. Erikson, 1965.

3. Winnicott sees this 'subjective object' as playing a necessary role in establishing the child's view of the independent reality of his mother, who up to now has existed solely as a fantasized object subject to the force of his emotions, and consequently in considerable danger of being destroyed by his anger. In the form of whatever he has chosen to be his 'transitional object', however, Mother has something approaching an independent life: he can vent his fury on her without destroying her. He can even kill her and bring her back to life again. He is on the way to learning to cope with 'things out there'.

4. They are found in Mary Shelley's *Frankenstein*, Oscar Wilde's *The Fisherman and His Soul*, R. L. Stevenson's *Dr Jekyll and Mr Hyde*, von Chamisso's *Peter Schlemihl*, Hermann Hesse's *Steppenwolf*, Aldous Huxley's *Grey Eminence*, Goethe's *Faust* and Shakespeare's *Tempest* (for Caliban).

5. Jung is careful to point out that the archetypes are in no way a product of imagination. On the contrary they represent 'a mental precondition and a characteristic of the cerebral function' (1938: 112).

6. C. G. Jung, *Psychology and Alchemy*, Collected Works, R.K.P., 1953: 462. 'On the Relation of Analytical Psychology to Poetic Art', *Contributions to Analytical Psychology*, (trans. H. G. & C. E. Baynes) London 1928.

7. Shamanism – 'A religion of Siberian tribes involving belief in secondary gods and in the power of shamans or priests to influence these.' OED. In fact, shamanism spreads far beyond Siberia, and its imagery has an universal significance.

8. A construct is like a reference axis, a basic dimension of appraisal, often unverbalised, frequently unsymbolized, and occasionally unsignified in any manner except by the elemental processes it governs. Behaviourally it can be regarded as an open channel of movement, and a system of constructs provides each man with his own personal network of action pathways, serving both to limit his movements and to open up to him passages of freedom which otherwise would be psychologically non-existent' (1955: 199).

Chapter 3

Drama and Depression

The connection between clinical depression and the urge to take part in drama may not at first be obvious, but is nonetheless, I believe, a real one. In this chapter we shall be comparing some aspects of depression with what we have already noticed of the ways in which theatre functions.

Over-tight construing has been associated with a tendency towards anxiety in that it is a defensive ploy by means of which a person tries to keep the tightest hold of what is going on without having to face the possibility of having to change his view of himself and the world. It is always the world that changes, never himself. This is also the kind of awareness found in depressed people, but with an important difference. The research of Bannister (1960) showed that, in depression, a swing occurs within a previously stable system: 'a sudden invalidation of one or two major superordinates within a construct system, producing a tendency for parts of the system to become weak.' Constructs contained in this part of the system were loosely related, while everything else remained as tightly organised as before. In addition to the dimensions of 'looseness' and 'tightness' in construing, there is also one of 'variability', associated mainly with depression.

Depressed people, then, may be prone to having the integrity of their construct systems suddenly destroyed. The effect of this is that a whole part of their world seems to fall away at their feet. Attending to whatever is contained in this part involves a crossing over into a gray area of uncertainty and this is an experience to which they are unaccustomed, having enjoyed the benefits of a self-protective tightness so successfully for so long. A loosely construing individual might not find the experience so painful. The depressive, however, has firmly embraced one way of dealing with life's problems: an effective way for most things that happen, but certainly not flexible enough to accommodate the effects of real trauma. Now he is left in the ambiguous territory between two ways of being, and it is a terrain for which he is singularly ill-equipped. No wonder he is angry, both with himself and other people. It is within this particular area, that of our relationship with others, that the integrity, or lack of it, of our construct system is most important. It is a *personal* construct system, and its subject matter as well as its *modus operandi* are concerned with what occurs among people. In the case of depression, someone who was sure about his or her relationship with other people is sure no longer, and hovers between hope and despair, striving to recapture the sense of belonging that they enjoyed before their image of themselves was shattered. The powerful feelings engendered by depression originate in a state of affairs according to which the self becomes 'stuck' in a single view of itself. As with schizophrenia, a particular way of trying to make sense of people and events has been driven home to the exclusion of all others. Investigation of the construct systems of depressed people reveals them to be organised in ways that lack flexibility, and dominated by a limited range of powerful ideas which permeate every area of thought, particularly those connected with the person him or herself: what Kelly calls 'pre-emptive core constructs'. This means that the self is always construed in terms of the same handful of ideas – good–bad, strong–weak, innocent–guilty, lovable–unlovable, the emphasis always being on the negative pole. Rather than experimenting with alternative ways of construing an expanding range of experiences, depressed people avoid anxiety by constricting their perceptual field to exclude events that are not easily contained within their existing range of constructs (1955: 477). How this has happened is open to argument; but it seems likely that such an approach has been learned, and that these dominant constructs have been locked into the system by their repeated use as a way of coping with life. Dorothy Rowe concludes that 'This way of seeing oneself and the world does not come into being overnight. It begins with young children having those experiences which teach them to construe themselves as bad. Sometimes children learn this through other people's definitions: 'What a bad boy you are', 'You really are an evil little girl'. More often the child decides to see himself or herself as bad rather than endure the greater peril of knowing that the people on whom his safety depends cannot be trusted. 'My good mother punishes me because I'm bad' (1985: 151). Our self-understanding is continually being validated by people who accept our own view of ourselves, particularly when this accords with their own ways of construing us. The experiences are repeated, the prophecies fulfilled, and the natural ability to deal with new situations in ways that are new – to alternate our constructs – begins to decay.

Because the number of available constructs about the self is limited, it is less possible to 'think round' the self-punitive attitude of mind that sees itself as confined to the negative pole of all available ways of looking at life. This, in fact, explains why depressed people are so vulnerable to shifts of mood. They are driven by the lack of alternative ways of construing to take refuge at the other pole of the same construct in which they are imprisoned. Instead of thinking and feeling in an alternative way, using different poles of reference (constructs), a depressed person veers wildly to the contrasting position within the same scale. Kelly describes this as 'slot-rattling'; it makes nonsense of the way in which an individual interprets, and consequently anticipates, events. Rather, it is a panic attempt to avoid the psychic pain involved in being imprisoned at the negative pole of a pre-emptive core construct. Unfortunately, the importance of the construct means that its invalidation in this way 'implies dislodgement of the core role structure' – a person's fundamental understanding about him or herself – 'so that a consistent and stable sense of well being cannot be maintained over time' (Ross, 1985: 166).

The result of this seemingly automatic tendency to shift backwards and forwards between the opposite poles of a single construct is a deadening feeling of confinement within the self, in which one is both jailer and jailed. Perhaps this is why, when things go wrong, depressed people tend easily to give up hope. How long this sense of helplessness lasts depends, of course, on the individual concerned. In cases of bi-polar depression it may be followed by a more or less rapid swing back into confidence and elation, but people with depressed personalities are likely to have a generally lowered mood most of the time. They feel that they are the victims of their own feelings – whether these originate in themselves, or are reflected upon them by others – and have very little sense of real autonomy, believing that their involvement in any enterprise is likely to be to the disadvantage of all concerned.

There is reason to believe that this should not be taken at face value, however. Depressed people are as aware of the faults of others as other people are, but instead of directing their annoyance against whomever it is that offends them, they turn it inwards upon themselves. In situations where other people act purposefully and creatively to change the environment, depressives torture themselves, going to considerable efforts to present as convincing a picture as they possibly can of their own personal worthlessness and guilt. The cognitive psychologist A. T. Beck distinguishes three characteristics of depression: a negative view of the self, a negative expectation of the future, and a tendency to screen out positive factors in one's awareness, so that only negative elements in a situation are construed as having any significance (1961).

In fact, such people are much less inadequate than they seem. The task of the psychotherapist, says Anthony Storr, 'is not only to reinforce the glimmer of hope which has brought the patient to seek help, but also to disinter the active aggressive aspect of his personality which, being largely repressed, is unavailable to him' (1979: 95). The kind of supportive relationship associated with psychotherapy may be of great help to depressed people. The origin of their condition is to be found in the first relationships they knew; however painful and damaging the experience which actually brought them to seek help – a bereavement, the loss of a precious job, a broken love affair – it seems out of proportion to the despair induced by it. Something else, a fact of even profounder significance to the personality of the depressed man or woman, lies at the bottom of all this negativity and hopelessness, this tendency to cling on to their own despair.

We are entitled to ask what this may be. Why has a depressed person so little self-esteem? Why has he or she never learned to cope with the tragedies of living? When we are born we are almost totally helpless, completely dependent on the ministrations of other people. We do not know what we can or cannot do. As we grow older we are still dependent, for much longer than any other animal. With increasing maturity comes awareness of the degree to which we depend on adults, and how inferior our capabilities are in comparison with theirs. If we are lucky enough to enjoy a high degree of validation as individuals — what Winnicott called 'good enough mothering' — and we are cuddled, played with, made to feel that we are contributing in a valuable way to whatever is going on within the family group, the sense of being dependent and inferior is countered by repetitive experiences of being made to feel important and whole. Our parents are no longer oppressive rivals but close friends, and admirers. If, throughout our childhood, each achievement is praised in a special personal way, in order to bring home the value placed on *us*, we will come to believe in the truthfulness of our parents' good opinions.

Thus, the child comes to think highly of itself because its parents obviously value its achievements and its own personal worth. This is an ordinary sort of thing to happen. In fact it is normal human behaviour. If it goes wrong the child suffers. Children are not spoken to and played with; they are kept in a dependent state, treated as beloved objects rather than contributing members of a family. Parents set standards which are so high that children are permanently discouraged; they have been continually tested, and have continually failed. The argument has been proved: this person is worthless. This kind of experience may be the origin of guilt feelings which are out of proportion to any actual rule-breaking on the part of the child. If parent-figures are consistently disapproving, there is little chance of a child growing up with any real self-respect. As she (or he) is bound to identify with the adults closest to her, guilt is almost compulsory. In particular, the closer the relationship to the mother figure, the one directly involved in the nurturing process, the more powerful the implication of personal guilt. This is because the child is bound to take upon itself the mother's condemnation of unacceptable behaviour: she rejects it, and so must I, even if in doing so I reject myself in the process. There is nothing abnormal in this. As we saw, infants are bound to identify, and mothers to show disapproval of unacceptable behaviour. The ensuing guilt-feelings are repressed as the guiding principle of consciousness, the ego, develops the strength to reject them as both unreasonable in themselves and counter-productive for the business of living. In most cases, the experience of being criticised or judged is outweighed by the knowledge that love is indeed present, so that punitive (and consequently self-punitive) events are incidental rather than characteristic, and that the child feels secure and appreciated. It is only where consistent or habitual de-valuing is the rule that the process we have described takes place, and the child grows into maturity in an emotionally handicapped condition, crippled by chronic feelings of guilt and unworthiness.

In fact, of course, there is no sense in which such a state of being can be called 'maturity'. Deprived at an early age of essential resources of love and security that he or she will need for the journey through life, particularly of the kind of relationship with others which is experienced as a validation of self rather than criticism and condemnation, a person is prevented from achieving the condition we call maturity. To be mature is to possess integrity of personhood – to know who one is, and to value oneself for being precisely that person. Eric Fromm describes a type of immature personality which he calls the 'receptive' character. People like this fit this specification very well indeed. They see themselves as perpetually taking, rarely giving, in the sense of making a real contribution to the relationships which involve them. Everything they need from life is located outside themselves. Security, expertise, understanding are only to be gained from others, so that any successes they achieve in life are never their own, but always the result of their having been fortunate enough one way or another to receive help from someone else. Such a person habitually presents him or herself as inadequate for the task in hand, for in this way they can fulfil several aims at once: awaken other people's protective instincts, give them the satisfaction of demonstrating their own superior abilities, and avoid having to make any real effort themselves. In this way they circumvent the kind of life-experience, painful but psychologically necessary, that might in itself contribute to the growth of their own maturity. Certainly, when he or she knows that there is somebody to look after them, the receptive character is relaxed, friendly, and responsive. What he or she craves is reassurance. Why they crave it is because of a chronic sense of inadequacy and insecurity founded in a very deep suspicion that they are, after all, fundamentally unacceptable to others.

Inadequacy, rejection, guilt, resentment and suppressed anger. These, of course, are feelings associated with depression. From childhood, the depressed individual is locked into a situation in which he or she must receive approbation without ever believing in its sincerity. As Storr says 'repeated assurance of good opinion is as necessary to his psychic health as are repeated feeds of milk to the physical well-being of infants' (1979: 99). Freud refers to depressive personalities as being fixated at the 'oral' stage; they feed on the approval of others and are so painfully dependent on what people think of them that they dare not run the risk of offending anybody. Their need is aggressive, their behaviour over-submissive. Their awareness of others makes them sensitive to the feelings and intentions of those around them without being able to contribute in a positive way to the relationships in which they are involved. Strong on empathy, they are weak on responsiveness, having, they feel, so little to give in exchange.

Others see depression in a more hopeful light, as the frustration of a powerful creativity. From a personal construct point of view, depressives may be regarded as frustrated artists. Kelly's 'creativity cycle' starts with 'loosened construction' and ends in construction that has been 'tightened', and consequently validated. In other words, in order to think in a creative way we review all the possibilities in as free and unconstrained a manner as we can, before deciding on a particular idea or course of action and committing ourselves to it, focusing in on it in the hope that it will 'work'. If it does, our interpretation of the state of affairs is, temporarily at least, validated. *We* are validated. This happens in and through an assertion of creativity. Art itself is the manipulation of distance to allow changes to take place in the way we 'see' the world; but it only works if we are willing to give it the life of our own creativity. George Kelly based his system of 'fixed role therapy' on the co-operation of people whose construct systems had been deliberately loosened by processes designed to free the imagination and make it possible for them to leave the old way of seeing the world and themselves, and invest in a new one.

As may be imagined, a good deal of ourselves goes into this kind of adventure, and when it fails to come off the result may be very discouraging – hence the view of depression as originating in 'tightened and *in*validated construing' (Jones, 1985: 171). Like Seligman's dogs, we have laid our safety on the line once too often.[1] Aesthetic distance communicates responsibility as well as freedom; standing back to see more clearly, we give ourselves in the seeing. We are not always wise, not always successful. At least part of the pain of depression is the agony of defeat. If we are defeated too often, we give up trying.

Anthony Storr has written extensively about the relationship between depression and creativity, drawing attention to the ways in which the second may help to alleviate the effects of the first. If a person is both talented and fortunate – fortunate enough, that is, to be widely regarded as a creative artist – the esteem of others, repeatedly expressed, may have the effect of convincing him or her that he or she possesses actual value in their eyes. The evidence is there, and it is evidence of a tangible kind; the books are read, the pictures looked at, the music played and heard. This is not mere reassurance, but objective proof, and as such it must have very real value for someone of low self-esteem. This is not to say that the evidence is always felt to be entirely convincing, even in the case of an artist with a considerable reputation (or even an internationally famous one, like Tchaikovsky, for instance). As Storr says 'one feature of this type of psychopathology is that the effect of the infection does not last. Success does bring self-esteem, reassurance, and even elation to the depressive; but the improvement is generally short-lived. In the end, no amount of external success compensates for what has not been incorporated in early childhood' (1972: 105). Extensive creative activity requires months or even years of persistent effort, the kind of thing which depressed people find hard, or even impossible, simply because they have never believed that their work can really merit such intense application; when people say it does they tend to think they are being flattered or appeased – people are simply being kind to them, they don't deserve it. Artists like this are often under-achievers, preferring quick rewards because they find it hard to stick at anything long enough to convince others or themselves of their real ability. Because they are trying to please other people rather than to satisfy their own creative instincts they end up doing neither very well, and so forfeit the opportunity for genuine self-expression which their talent holds out to them. The intention is to placate, rather than create.

Genuine artists, on the other hand, give of themselves in order to look at what they have made. He – or she – is object-centred, inviting other people to enter their world. Instead of setting out to explore territory which is already shared, already common property, an artist's work reveals himself, his or her own unique world. To do this is to assert selfhood in the strongest, most dramatic way, by shattering the world which has been received from others and restructuring it in ways that are uniquely their own. To shatter the world of other people is not enough. Somehow a connection must be made, a bridge built, between self and other by which the self's *creative acceptability*, its ability to win an unique kind of personal acceptance on its own terms, is established.

Thus, far from being simply a means of self-expression, an artist's work calls forth love from other people. The form that this takes is that of a loving respect. This is precisely the kind of love originally needed for the eventual achievement of emotional maturity, the missing ingredient, in fact, from the artist's childhood experience. The effect may be diffuse, but the underlying process is the same, each successive act of creation representing a new attempt to lay hold of an elusive security of relationship between the artist and other people. Certainly, not all artists function in this one-sided fashion. You do not have to be an immature person, searching for ways of compensating for half-remembered humiliations, fighting over and over again battles which can never be won, to create beauty for your own and others' enjoyment. Nevertheless, the work of psychologists and psycho-analysts, and the testimony of artists themselves, provides evidence which leads us to suspect that a creative person may feel a particularly strong need for the validation which proceeds from the responsiveness of others. Only this, it seems, can bring something of the sense of personal wholeness of which the artist feels deprived.

What, then, is the connection between the reality the artist creates with the express intention of sharing it with others, and the received reality of other people? It is not the straightforward division of subjective and objective, the artist's subjectivity and the objectivity of others affected by it; nor is it the coming together of two subjectivities, although it might well be thought to be this. What happens involves an expansion of the total world of interpersonal experience, the creation of something genuinely new, a new way of breaking down the subjective–objective division. The inspiration and the impulse proceed from the artist, but from communication rather than simple self-expression To a certain extent it is an aggressive gesture. Indeed, in many people considered to be of a depressive personality there is a manic element at war with the need to win approval which we have recognised as a main characteristic of depression. This tendency is in fact the opposite of depression. It cries out to be heard in an effort to dominate the environment and subdue everything within it that might reduce the self to dependency and self-loathing. This is the well established 'manic-depressive psychosis'. It is associated with creativeness in a great many cases, and many famous artists have suffered from it, to their personal sorrow and civilization's lasting glory. In such cases the pain of an intensive subjectivity can only be assuaged by an activity able to transform the entire world for those who live in it.[2]

One thing above all needs to be stressed. This reaching out to public reality requires courage. It is the opposite of the lack of self-confidence which characterizes depressed states. It is not simply a question of mood-swings. What is important here from our point of view is the *content* of the mood. From their dialectical experience of the world manic-depressive people find the spiritual strength to surpass what they see around them and to create something new. There is no desire to confine the self to the exploration of personal reality; rising to the occasion, they assault the world that conspires to reduce them. Whereas schizoid people concentrate upon whatever it is that is going on 'inside' them, manic-depressives seek to reduce confusion in the outside world to achieve a kind of mastery over whatever faces them. In their private lives they tend towards sociability, enjoying the presence of other people in the manic phase, looking to them for comfort and support when depressed.

In my own experience within the theatre, I have gained an impression that those actors who incline towards a depressed emotional tone find that acting before an audience has an invigorating effect. It may be that this is one of the reasons why they became actors in the first place. If so, it makes a kind of sense, for the experience of theatre hovers between involvement with and separation from others, specifically designed in its balance of contrivance and spontaneity to make the adventure of involvement as safe as possible without lessening its force. For all who lack self-confidence but can overcome their initial stage fright to the point of actually setting foot on stage, the theatre extends a warm welcome: for those who are depressed it provides an experience of acceptance which, for a time at least gives them the courage they need both for the play itself and for life. This is a mediated acceptance, because the performer is 'in role', and therefore distanced from the source of the emotion that inspires him or her. On stage it is possible to enjoy the reality of human relationship at one remove and still benefit from it.

In fact, sociologists who make use of the dramaturgical model to analyse human interaction employ the metaphor of aesthetic distance to describe types of personality from the point of view of their relational aspects. An 'over-distanced' individual, for example, customarily functions in a detached way towards others: he or she is a private kind of person, one who does not easily share experiences, and presents an unemotional face to the world. Typically, he or she prefers ideas to experiences, functioning intellectually rather than instinctively or intuitively. A person diagnosed as schizophrenic would almost certainly be of this type. On the other hand, people who are 'under-distanced', given the chance, behave in the opposite way. Their desire to find relief in self-exposure leads them to act in ways which the rules determining appropriate behaviour in social situations usually designate as over-personal. These are the people who whisper loud comments in church; at relaxed gatherings they tend to exploit brief acquaintanceships as if they were long-standing friendships, embarrassing old friends with remarks which are 'too near the bone', in their desire for contact. In other words their behaviour is considered to be too socially demanding, and to lack the necessary distance between persons upon which the smooth functioning of social groups depends.

The connection between 'under-distancing' and the experience of people who tend to suffer from periods of depression is a striking one. Both kinds of people demand constant reassurance from others that they are valued, appreciated, loved; both kinds will go out of their way to get it, and both will appear to be utterly unconvinced that they have in fact got the regard for which they hunger and thirst. The spontaneity of their self-giving, coupled with that talent for empathic understanding which comes from the need to assimilate, and so disarm, the other person, may awaken a very genuine love, a whole-hearted appreciation and respect, on the part of people who really know them. Indeed, they may be generally regarded as admirable members of society because of these things. It does not matter to them, however. Nothing is enough to satisfy the need for reassurance which opens up like a chasm inside them whenever they turn their thoughts to themselves and what they believe to be their 'true' condition.

At this level of analysis, then, depression and lack of social distance are associated, in that both imply a desire for an unattainable degree of contact with other people, an involvement which is deep enough to assuage the profoundest need for personal authentification; both receive love but cannot identify themselves as people who are themselves loved, giving love in ways which may be experienced as overpowering by those in receipt of them; both demand a degree of attention from others which can never be satisfied, while devoting most of their own attention to themselves in the effort to gauge just how acceptable, how close to others, they in fact are. The actor who is depressed, whose personal life lacks distance, gains spiritual strength by exposing him-or herself to others in a special way, sharing his or her fantasies with the audience under the guise of the character in the play, receiving the gift of love from the audience in the shape of their imaginative participation in his or her performance. In this way I reveal enough of myself as I choose in the mode that I choose; I display my personality, or certain aspects of it, while safeguarding my true identity from the possibility of criticism or actual rejection.

In fact the actor achieves a closer contact than he or she may have expected. The illusion of theatre permits a degree of relationship which is more intense, more personal, than the calculated self-disclosure whereby the stage-performer uses his or her character as a disguise which permits selected aspects of the self to emerge. The actor's mask reveals more than he or she might at first suppose. As we saw, aesthetic distance promotes involvement rather than inhibiting it. What the under-distanced individual craves is not total immersion in another's being. What such a person is searching for, semi-consciously, is a way to be freed from what is felt to be a slavish dependence on the other's regard. Involvement to achieve autonomy is sought, the self-confidence that should have been gained during those early years of personal development and which has been looked for ever since, but which is always elusive however hard he or she tries to take hold of it. It is the lack of this that causes him or her to hate themselves publicly, and other people – the people they go out of their way to appear to love – in private. Release from his or her problems of human relationship are found within the drama. Protected by the contrived nature of the play we can stand back *as ourselves* while remaining in relationship with the other people involved, both actors and audience. In other words, the character which we have laboured so hard to make our own is free to live in the shared world of the story without any diminution of self.

The benefit of this for someone who tends towards depression is obvious. As we saw, depressed people tend to immerse themselves in the experience of others, without feeling free, or confident, enough to respond to that experience in a relationship of reciprocity and mutual concern. Response to the other requires distance between selves, if only because it is necessary to have an identifiable position to respond *from*. Theatre and drama provide such positions within a well-defined scenario of human interaction; drama therapy is largely based on the purposeful manipulation of aesthetic distance, carried out to allow those involved the freedom to experiment with their own image of themselves especially with regard to the crucial boundary between self and other. It is not surprising that depressed people are eager to take advantage of the opportunity to 'fit in' in this way, for the ability to give and receive more effectively is what they secretly crave. Above all, they need to find a way of sharing. The play provides ways which are safe and adventurous, opening up a universe of imaginative possibility which the experience of a genuine focused involvement renders experientially viable.

All this is inherent in the unique flexibility and expressiveness of drama as an art form. Each play represents a novel attempt at organising the countless imaginable ways in which men and women may relate to one another, with all the opportunities for re-interpreting our own experience that such a re-organisation offers. Its effect is to break the links which bind present and past in the world outside, loosening their power to limit our freedom. It is a place and time of new conclusions for old arguments, one in which long-lasting pre-occupations are laid aside. This distancing effect provides actors and audiences with a means of withdrawing from the world of relationships which sometimes threatens to swamp them, without withdrawing from, or diminishing in any way, their actual relationship with that world. The presence within the same context of a powerful feeling of involvement and a vivid new understanding of the way in which people and events, including oneself, interact brings an experience of wholeness to divided sensibilities. Actors' imagination leads them to seek out others with a view to putting together a scenario in which experiences may be exchanged, and developments occur, in ways which are adventurous and yet comparatively safe.

It is not the need to re-enact well-rehearsed scenes that attracts them so much as the sense of newness and possibility within the play. Things need to be lived out, not simply thought through. There is the need to act out ideas and emotions in an embodied way; to *interact with* people rather than simply act towards them. The genuinely dramatic character of drama therapy is guaranteed by the adoption of a truly contextual approach to human experience. Drama, and drama therapy may give rise to ideas, but they are *about* presences; presences which embody ideas. People are presented *in situ*, and our attention is directed to what is happening here and now, 'in the flesh'. As Sue Jennings says 'for his mental, physical and emotional well-being, man has to rediscover his cultural roots by actually experiencing them in some form, *and being able to recreate them himself and not just observe this from others*'.[3] She goes on to say that 'the most important medium for this is man's own body' (1983: 49). This has been mentioned already, but needs specific attention with regard to depression. We have a natural ability to use our bodies rhythmically which is expressed in the ways we play, work, worship. If this is not given due expression we lose touch with a fundamental dimension of our humanity. In an over intellectualized society men and women are in danger of losing touch with themselves at the most basic level. This is the level of 'body awareness', the experience of *having a body at all*, which precedes 'body image', or the way we are accustomed to regard our own bodies. Body awareness allows us to distinguish ourselves from other people at a level which gives rise to the first stirrings of that social life which will sustain us as human beings. In order to relate to others I must have a real sense of myself as an embodied entity, a definite organism, to be bestowed or retained at my own will. The subjective experience of individuals within society, their body image, is dependent upon the objective presence of social structure, for the mechanism of perception itself makes use of the primitive relational categories provided by the embodied human environment.[4] Movement, dance, drama, team games, underlie the specifically therapeutic uses of bodily experience, involving a somatic interaction which provides expression and release for depressed people at a level preceding cognition, the level of bodily union and interdependence associated with the courage to be human.

This is not to be confused with movement which is strictly regulated or 'drilled' so as to produce bodily skills of a high degree of sophistication to be deployed first of all self-consciously, then automatically. What concerns us here is movement and gesture used expressively in ways that are spontaneous and expressive, owing more to feeling than to thought. At the same time the element of form is present, which provides a framework of safety within which instinct can be allowed to flourish. This is not so much a set of rules to be applied and remembered as the semi-conscious awareness that what is happening is within a particular context which may be taken for granted and need not be studiously recalled.

As Kretschmer pointed out, depressed people are often of a stocky build, the kind of figure that often 'runs to fat', quite unlike the athletic physique associated with actors. One would not think that an actor with such a personality would feel at home on stage. Surely he or she would feel self-conscious in front of so many people! And yet they do not seem to feel anything of the kind. More often than not they seem to enjoy the play, attacking their parts with gusto. So far as I can see there are two reasons for this. The first concerns the feeling of security that actors experience when they are 'playing a part', in spite of the extreme state of arousal caused by the presence of the audience – the emotional focusing we noticed earlier on. The issues of the play are simpler than those of life, its reasons clearer and more direct. They affect the depressed person with the force of meaning set free from reflection. The second reason, which is even more important, is the power of the creative imagination. Whatever a player feels on stage is not directly concerned with his or her own personal characteristics, but with those of the character being acted and the play being performed. By concentrating on the part the player is protected and exposed – exposed at an emotional level but protected from self-consciousness. Physical factors contribute to this too. Among these are the significance of gesture and posture, the *tempi* of action and reaction, the intonation of speech, all contributing to the physical 'shape' of the play. These might be called the play's 'action-linkages', for they all contribute to the satisfaction involved in creating a world and sharing it with others.

On the other hand, depressed people control their own weight in accordance with their own undervalued self-image. Both anorexia and obesity are connected with depression, which is sometimes expressed in over-eating, sometimes by not eating enough. The way we react to our depression varies according to whether we are trying to comfort or to punish ourselves – a good example of the interplay of action and reaction within the whole sphere of human psychology. In the next chapter, we shall see how the approach that helps untie psychological knots can also give shape to ideas that are too loosely constructed to be useful as signposts for action in the world, as drama combines 'loosening' and 'tightening' within the same experience.

Notes

1. In a series of experiments with dogs, M. E. P. Seligman showed that persistent failure to solve a problem – how to reach food without receiving an electric shock – had the effect of inducing a state very like human depression, so that for a long time afterwards the dogs refused to perform well-rewarded tasks that were within their abilities. They appeared to have lost interest in responding to anything at all. Seligman calls this condition 'learned helplessness'.

2. Examples of manic depressive artists are very numerous. Among the more famous are Schumann, Tchaikovsky, Wolf.

3. My own italics.

4. As Durkheim and Mauss pointed out 'far from it being the case that the social relations of men are based on logical relations between things, in reality it is the former which have provided the prototype for the latter' (1963: 82).

Chapter 4

Drama and Schizophrenia
A Personal Construct Approach to Thought Disorder

'An individual', says Eric Fromm, 'may live among people and yet be overcome with an utter feeling of isolation, the outcome of which, if it transcends a certain limit is the state of insanity which schizophrenic disturbances represent' (1960: 15). In other words, other people do not simply have to be present, they have to be *real*. They cannot simply be our own inventions. Not only this, but we must be able to adapt our interpretation of reality time and time again in order to continue to be in communication with the world in which we live. This necessitates more than the re-arrangement of our 'mental furniture' to give plausibility to our own fantasies. We have to take real account of the demands of the outside world and try to fit in with it. Within certain limits we may choose how to react, but the outcome is rarely in our hands. Most of the time we are conscious of being enmeshed in a network of control and subordination in which self and not-self interact as part and parcel of the same process. Those who have never developed the ability to make systematic contact with a reality other than their own subjective one are not only lonely, but confused. Anthony Storr describes schizophrenic patients as 'trying to make sense out of an arbitrary and unpredictable universe' (1976: 110). They are like spectators at a football match who can only see one very limited section of the field and yet keep being expected to join in the game. Their inability to step outside themselves and observe the match from someone else's viewpoint means that they never know which angle the ball is coming from next. In *Playing and Reality*, Winnicott speaks of the impoverishment of a patient's life because of her inability to 'stand in the other person's shoes'. He suggests that 'a psycho-pathology of the schizoid states' might have much to gain from investigation into the part played by transitional objects in the development of the individual's ability to come to terms with other people's reality. Certainly, in making sense of our relationships with other people we give shape not only to our social life but to our experience of the world itself. The mechanism of perception itself makes use of the categories provided by the environment of other human beings, for people are by far the most important objects we perceive. They possess a different kind of reality from anything else and their relationships with one another provide a model for the associations and separations which we discern in our perception of the way that reality is put together. Ideas that originate in, and are fleshed-out by, personal relationships provide the foundation of our individual construct systems, the basis on which we put together our own individual argument about the meaning of life. In his investigations into schizophrenic thought-disorder, Bannister reached the conclusion that the ability to make sense of people was more affected by the condition than was the ability to organise things. As we saw in the last chapter, our relationship with people is the key to our world.[1]

If the significance of people as the structural elements around which perception is ordered is so great, it follows that the success with which we are able to construct our personal world will depend on the amount of co-operation we encounter on their part, particularly the co-operation of those within our immediate environment. Quality and consistency of mothering may not be all that is needed to help the child learn how to relate to others. However necessary it may be for the provision of the initial security the child needs to enable it to reach out beyond itself, once this stage has been reached something else must come into play. In other words, the 'transitional object' has two points of reference without which it cannot really function as it should. The transition involved is from security to security across the chasm of isolation and defencelessness: from the security of a state of affairs in which the self is everything, a strictly private world, to that of a universe of dependable relationships, people and situations that can be trusted *because the rules governing their behaviour can be learned*. Whereas the infant formerly trusted the world, and his own private core of sensation and activity within it, without distinction, now he must place his confidence in a group of people whose intentions towards and expectations of him he can construe in a satisfactory way. His world will never again be so complete, so perfect in its interior balance, but he will strive with the co-operation of others to construct a network of achievable meanings which will provide a measure of security and a purpose for living.

Obviously he cannot do this by himself. If the messages he receives from other people lack clarity, so that he can form no strong impressions about them, he will have difficulty in predicting their behaviour and selecting his own responses to it. If the information he receives is confused and self-contradictory, the world he constructs will share these characteristics. Even if he responds to rules of regularity and consistency perceivable in the world as a whole, and then tries hard to make sense of what he is offered by people, the struggle to process data which is self-contradictory is bound in the end to discourage him and to reduce his confidence in the accuracy of the predictions he makes.

Considerations of this kind lie behind theories of the 'schizogenic' family, which suggest that destructive family interactions are the cause of schizophrenia. These include the 'double bind' hypotheses of Bateson *et al* (1956), the view which relates schizophrenia to parental 'inculcation of confused and distorted meanings', presented by Lidz (1964, 1975), and arguments concerning the disintegrating effects of 'mystification' by forms of family process, as put forward by Laing and Esterson (1970).

(1) In the 'double bind' situation the person subjected to the 'bind' receives two separate and conflicting messages of a kind which cannot be ignored and where the contradiction is not self-evident. They are consequently faced with behaviour which invites two constructions, either of which will be invalidated and neither of which provides any basis for effective anticipation of ensuing events. An example might be 'I'm very happy for you' in a tone, or with a facial expression, which suggests the opposite.[2] Faced with this kind of contradictory communication over an extended period of time, an individual adapts either by withdrawing into a fantasy world in which thinking and feeling can be more straightforward (too straightforward in fact for learning to deal with reality), or by reproducing the same kind of ambiguity and irrationality in their own thinking and behaviour. Because they can never be right, they find a way of defending themselves by contriving never to be wrong. Like their mentors, they too will systematically disguise their intentions, so that they can never be held responsible for anything they say or do. Their confusing behaviour is a way of coping. Knowing that they can't understand their elders, they come up with a way, learnt from them, of hiding their failure from them – and also from themselves.

(2) Lidz expands Bateson's dual model into a threefold one, concentrating in particular upon the relationship between the parents, and the effect of this upon the child. Where there is a very definite imbalance in the way in which parents fulfil their roles towards the child a situation may develop in which he or she is subjected to a distorted view of the world imposed on him or her because it reflects the way in which the parents themselves view reality: 'The parents' delimitation of the environment and their insistence on altering the family members' perceptions and meanings, create a strange family milieu filled with inconsistencies, contradictory meanings, and a denial of what should be obvious' (1968: 179). Forced by their own inadequacy to sustain what Lidz describes elsewhere as 'parental coalition and proper maintenance of generation boundaries and gender roles' (1975: 21) – in other words a dependable structure of parental interaction – the parents present the child with a model of the world which is inherently confusing and, once again, self-contradictory. The model contradicts itself because it is obviously one kind of thing, yet claims to be something entirely different.[3]

That this kind of systematic destruction of inter-personal sense takes place within the families of patients diagnosed as schizophrenic has been claimed by several writers. Wynne and Singer (1963a and b) consider that the kinds of thought-disorder associated with schizophrenia originate in the way that the parents of schizophrenic children themselves speak and think. Because attempts at direct communication on the part of the children always fail, they develop a form of idiosyncratic pseudo-communication, in which they are really talking to themselves. In this way they are able to avoid the experience of being consistently mis-translated. Again, if they cannot 'be themselves' in public, growing and developing in a free relationship with their parents, they will nurture their identity in private. Unfortunately, however, this leads to a greater confusion as the self defines itself in and through its messages to the other.

(3) As we have seen, Object Relations Theory sees schizophrenia as originating in ontological insecurity and leading to existential confusion. Certainly there seems little doubt that failure in the business of making sense lies at the root of the schizophrenic condition. Laing and Esterson (1970), Cox (1978), and Bannister (1960, 1962B, 1965, 1966, 1975) lay great stress on the need to take the communications of people diagnosed as schizophrenic very seriously indeed, even when, (or particularly when), they are suffering from thought disorder. Laing and Esterson lay stress on the importance of trying to see what is going on within the social system of which the person defined as sick is a key part: much of what is customarily taken to be part of the symptomatology of an organic schizophrenic process, an identifiable mental illness, is 'intelligible as social praxis'. In other words, the difficulty concerns the way in which the people concerned are construing what is happening among them. Again, it is widely stated that the fact that they do not understand what is really going on is explicable because they have lost the ability to see things from one another's point of view, so that they repeatedly misinterpret one another's intentions. The ensuing 'mystification' need not be the result of one person's determination to disguise his or her own intentions, as in Lidz's model; it may be a genuine mistake about other people's intentions which gives rise to a whole succession of misinterpretations, spreading out like the ripples on a pond. As the confusion grows it centres around a particular member of the social nexus, who becomes the 'patient'. This individual is almost totally confounded by conflicting information about what other people say, what they mean, what they ought to mean, what they really mean, what he himself ought to mean, what he really wants to mean, what other people want him to mean, what he wants other people to want him to mean, etc. etc. It seems, then, that the first thing to do in all this is to try and find out what they themselves really mean; what they were trying to communicate before the exchange got jammed. The confused, fragmented, and

self-contradictory message represents their own attempt to make sense of a senseless situation. Somehow the link between the personal view and that of other people has become lost. All sets of views, say Laing and Esterson, must be rediscovered and clarified, and the connections reflected back upon those concerned for the benefit of the whole social nexus.

In terms of construct theory the breakdown of communication involved in schizophrenic thought-disorder means that an individual's personal constructs have been systematically prevented from forming a reliable system, so that all his attempts at building up a stable universe of expectations and reactions have foundered. Such an individual will never know what is likely to happen in the future, because so little up to now has ever turned out the way it was expected to. Don Bannister states the situation clearly: 'To construe a situation…is to predict future events, and if constructs are essentially predictions it follows that future events may either validate them, invalidate them or turn out to be 'irrelevant' – i.e. the events which follow the prediction prove to be outside the range of convenience of the constructs used to predict them' (1962B: 840). The effect of this 'serial invalidation', Bannister claims, is to make connections between constructs looser, so that they become less dependent on one another. If something no longer 'ties in' with something else, it cannot be used to predict its occurrence. However, although it 'can no longer generate stable, unidirectional predictions', it may be used in a vaguer, less definite way, as an explanation of things that have already happened.

This is obviously very important indeed. In a world where nothing definite is expected, nothing is ever a surprise. Understanding becomes a provisional thing, flexible enough to take account of any contingency. In this condition it is much less useful for constructing relationships, but causes people a good deal less anxiety because it is so much easier to make some kind of sense out of anything at all.[4] Thus Don Bannister: 'Schizophrenic thought-disorder is experienced subjectively as living in a fluid, unfocused and undifferentiated world in which anxiety is not felt to any marked degree since only the vaguest and least destructible anticipations arise in the mind of the subject' (1962b: 841). This is the 'loose construing' described by Kelly, according to which individual constructs lead to contradictory predictions, but manage to retain their own identity because they do not form part of any integrated network of meanings.

To sum up. For these writers, it is the breakdown of social relationships, or the failure to allow them to develop in the first place, that gives rise to schizophrenic thought-disorder. It is not the only explanation, of course; it pays little regard to chemical changes occurring in the brain, or inherited characteristics of the central nervous system. It throws more light on the experience of drama therapy than such explanations do, however. Working dramatherapeutically with thought-disordered people it is possible to see changes taking place – more awareness of other people, a greater ability to share rather than simply include, much less tendency to withdraw from social contact – all of which suggest that the kind of explanation put forward by Lidz, who sees schizophrenia as 'regression, for defensive reasons, to earlier phases of cognitive development' (1975: 54), may be close to the truth. Such a process would be essentially reversible. Perhaps drama therapy might help.

The characteristic which psychologists, psychiatrists and psycho-analysts seize upon is an absence of a coherent structure for interpersonal communication, and consequently, for human relationship. The relevance to drama, with its dependence on structure, is obvious. According to Bannister 'the thought-disordered schizophrenic is left occupying a fluid, undifferentiated, subjective universe' (1962B: 833). In a way that seems very similar to this, Object Relations Theory sees a connection between the undifferentiated awareness which is supposed – logically enough – to characterise the state of 'infantile narcissism', and the symptomatology of schizophrenia. Winnicott's 'transitional object' represents the developing psyche's first successful attempt at structuring the world in a meaningful way by adopting a position which is at least a little detached from preoccupation with the self. If for some reason – inadequate mothering, trauma in later life leading to regression, having to cope repeatedly with self-contradictory instructions, persistent invalidation of constructs, mystification, the presentation of irrational models of behaviour – this ability does not develop, the individual awareness remains too firmly centred upon, or rooted in, the organism for it to develop as genuine perception, involving the organisation and re-organisation of construct relationships to get to grips with the world. This may result in a pathological limitation of existential freedom and increase in vulnerability. If I can recognise no difference between myself and whatever I am thinking about, my thoughts are as precious as I am myself, and also as vulnerable. I cannot change my mind without changing my being. 'The schizophrenic patient, in brief, believes that he is the focal point of events that are unrelated or coincidental to his life. Category formation must remain limited or defective if the self intrudes into all categorizations' (Lidz, 1975: 11).

The original standpoint of Winnicott and Lidz is vastly different from that of Kelly and Bannister, but the notion of a thought-disordered person limiting the range of flexibility of his perceptual categories for defensive purposes is common to both Object Relations Theory and Personal Construct Theory. The latter draws attention to the need to safeguard oneself from the confusion contingent upon a chronic failure to predict events, while the former posits a self engaged in restricting its own area of vulnerability by closing down perceptual channels which may require adaption and change. Both describe an individual who is determined to avoid being taken unawares by a world which is unpredictable, and consequently uncontrollable, and has taken action to limit his communication with that world in a way which is drastic and effective.

If thought disorder is something which has been learned from other people, as Laing and Esterson and Lidz suggest, or something which has been invented to serve as a protective mechanism for use in relationships involving other people (Bateson, Bannister), it would seem likely that it is modifiable by new learning, or by new kinds of learning. Indeed this seems probable even if the condition originates in an inherited inability to use publicly accessible thought-forms, or to reject all kinds of social communication. People can learn new things even if, for constitutional reasons, they find the process extremely difficult. Lidz says: 'I believe that psychotherapy...forms the core of the treatment (of schizophrenia). The therapeutic relationship enables the patient to emerge from his disillusionment and despair and to begin to trust and relate again' (1975: 127). Although psychotherapists of the analytic school have tended to see the condition as a more or less straightforward regression to 'primary process thinking' (Winnicott, for example, described it as a neurotic condition), Lidz is very much aware of the confusion and complexity of the structures involved.[5] He sees much more going on in the way of sheer conceptual confusion than Winnicott, and stresses the need for the provision of a model of clear communication which will provide patient and therapist with a meeting place in which both may feel safe and secure together, and from which either may make forays into the territory of the other.

Transitional objects exist to provide this kind of model. If schizoid states represent a failure to share in the other (Winnicott 1971: 135), then such objects, which make use of a form of communication originally invented by the patient himself, are of obvious therapeutic value. The patient may play with a model of his own thought, experimenting with various possibilities which are not apparent to him until the ideas involved are externalised. Even more importantly, he may incorporate the thoughts of another person, or even other people, within his experiments. Like a child with a toy, he plays at what terrifies him and learns how to internalise his fear. Plays allow people to communicate because they permit interchange between two levels of human experience, fantasy and reality. The expression of fantasy may be frowned on by those engaged in inculcating 'a sense of reality', but here it plays a key role in providing the setting for real communication to take place. It also promotes perceptual clarity, because the action of setting apart a special area for playing is nothing less than that of publicly discriminating between two kinds of reality and holding them in a creative tension with each other, so that neither is allowed to take on the characteristics of the other, but both may be used as ways of making sense of the world.

David Read Johnson draws attention to the importance of the setting in which therapy takes place: 'the therapeutic goal is to reverse...the vicious circle of primary boundary confusion, anxiety, and retreat from reality. Clearly an environment is needed in which relationship with others will be as non-threatening as possible, one with distinct boundaries and structure to insure that the insecure personality will not be engulfed. An environment must be created in which something of the inner self can be safely expressed, so that it can be identified and later integrated with the other parts of the self that have been cut off from it' (1981B: 50, 51). For each of these writers, the process of therapy depends on the establishment of authentic communication between patient and therapist. With communication comes structure, as individuals acknowledge the primary categories of 'self' and 'other' as a basis for more extensive differentiations. As Cox points out the environment itself may be structured to promote a feeling of safety and confidence (Cox, 1978).

Laing and Esterson concentrate entirely upon dealing as demystification. People who fear rejection may adopt a form of communication which disguises its true meaning, and needs to be specially interpreted. This serves a double purpose – I do not have to take full responsibility for having committed myself to actually meaning something, while you have to prove your goodwill towards me by working specially hard to understand me. The danger is that I may go on doing this after you have given up; particularly if it expresses how I feel about life. Laing and Esterson suggest that what the patient says is to be taken seriously as a *statement* rather than a *symptom*. If it seems confused or self-contradictory, then that is precisely what the patient means. The confusion often turns out to involve the literal use of metaphor, in which homology is used instead of analogy; instead of referring to something felt inwardly in terms of an object perceived or imagined outside oneself, both the experience and its referent occur 'within' the self. Reflected back by a therapist who is concentrating on making sense of what the patient is saying, the communication now refers to something in the outside world. One kind of reality is brought into relation with another, and the crucial distinction between inner and outer, the armature we use to make sense of the world, is re-established.

This is a fundamental consideration. It does not seem to be possible to organise one's perceiving of people in a way that is wholly solipsistic. Schizophrenic patients, certainly, reveal a need to communicate with other people. In the case of people with marked thought-disorder there is a desire to talk and be sociable, often increased by the inability of the people whom they are addressing to make sense of what they are saying. There is a process going on which involves the intermeshing of two ways of construing the world. The trouble is that the guide lines keep diverging so that both have the experience of 'going off the track' from time to time. On such occasions, thought-disordered people don't seem to see the necessity to 'stick to the point'. Despite a lack of encouragement at this linguistic level, the thought-disordered person remains interested in carrying on the conversation. His or her communication is odd, but it is *still communication*.

Those involved in psychotherapy sometimes stress the point that 'private' languages serve a double function, that of confusion and enticement (Grainger, 1979; Cox 1978). The need for communication is still there, but relationship has proved so painful in the past that other people must prove their goodwill by being willing to work out what the wounded person's message is. The question is whether this withdrawal into unintelligibility is deliberate or not. In the setting provided by a structured psychotherapeutic relationship the use of expressions and images which possess a meaning known only to oneself may be a kind of self-disclosure: 'This is too difficult for me to say. See if you are concerned enough to work it out for yourself!' The authorised ambiguity of drama is ideal for this kind of communication.

This is rather different from the situation of those who are established in thought-disorder and cannot be shocked out of it by a sudden inspirational interpretation on the part of the therapist in the safety of the therapeutic interview or the charmed circle of the group. If people become thought-disordered because of a breakdown in communication involving a defensive withdrawal from public reality it is unlikely, if not impossible, that they will suddenly snap back into normal ways of communicating. Because the development of the condition must have involved some kind of systematic re-structuring of the ways in which the world makes sense for the individual involved (it takes quite a long time to learn a language, even if it is to be used for talking only to yourself) any attempt to cure it must be equally painstaking. What has been learned must somehow be unlearned, and this can only be done by learning something new to take its place.

One approach which takes this into account is that of Don Bannister and his associates, the psychologists associated with him in his research. This is an application of Personal Construct Psychology. The gap between the thought disordered person and his environment of people and things is located within the organisation of his own personal construct system. Close engagement with the environment, openness to its influences and involvement in its on-going life, necessitate a tightly organised system for predicting and controlling it. If, over a long period of time and in a systematic way, the environment turns out to be both unpredictable and uncontrollable, evading all attempts to come to grips with it, an individual may find himself deeply discouraged. He will no longer try to make sense of life; there is nothing to make sense of. He will no longer expect to understand or be understood. In fact, so far as other people are concerned, he will no longer be surprised by anything that happens. The idea that some things 'tied in with one another' when compared to others has proved illusory once too often. From now on he will tend to construe each event separately, drawing as few conclusions about its relationship with other events as possible. Thus the pathological inclusiveness of self and other described by Object Relations Theory is reproduced here by a withdrawal of personal investment in interpersonal reality – an impersonal world which controls without ever being controlled.

   Construct theory rests upon the proposition that ideas 'hang together' in a trustworthy way because people's behaviour is consistent. If people behave inconsistently the thinking which they induce will lose its articulation, because the sense we make of life demands continual validation from the people and events we base it on. Thus, confused experience of relationship is, at its most fundamental level, the same thing as confused thinking. And when our ideas begin to lose their coherence this is because for us, other people have begun to 'come apart'. When they no longer conform to the model we have of reality, the model itself loses its precise definition. At this point Kelly suggests that we tend to make our model more vague in order to preserve its identity as a model of reality: reality is blurred, so our model is imprecise. Unfortunately it may become too inexact to function as a means of communication with the world of people and events it is intended to represent. The task of therapy is to provide evidence of the world's conformity to the individual's model, thus validating his constructs. Because his disordered thinking is primarily concerned with the way he construes people (Bannister and Salmon 1966), it must be done personally; because it is the result of experience over a considerable time, it must be done systematically.[6]

   In experiments involving normal subjects, it was shown that repeated validation led to a significant rise in the level of intercorrelation between constructs. Corroboration of one part of an individual's mental 'plan' had the effect of integrating the entire structure by vindicating its overall effectiveness as a way of predicting events. In other words, a person's ability to make consistent sense of the world increased whenever their attempts to do so turned out the way that they expected. Where constructs were systematically made to appear inappropriate (i.e. 'invalidated'), or where no information at all was given, the pattern of relationships between ideas changed in a marked way, losing its consistency, and consequently its ability to anticipate events efficiently. A certain amount of evidence was forthcoming which showed that such invalidation had led to loosened construing, but not at the level which had been found in thought-disordered schizophrenics. Later, however, Bannister and his associates carried out a study aimed at reversing the process of thought disorder by working with schizophrenic patients themselves: 'the construct system of each patient was extensively examined so as to try and locate clusters which however weakly they were related, were structured relative to the very loose system of which they were a part. The search was for islands of meaning in the generally chaotic and poorly structured fabric of the system of constructs which the patient used for viewing himself and other people in interpersonal and psychological terms' (1975: 172).

The approach followed here was significantly different from that of the previous experiment, a good deal of effort being put into the attempt to allow the patient to make his or her own kind of sense of whatever was going on within the experimental situation. This meant creating a special kind of interpersonal environment, one which was different from the world 'outside': 'it was hoped that as his construct system strengthened and elaborated in response to the construct environment, it would reach a point at which it was capable of surviving the *mixture* of validation and invalidation which the patient would inevitably experience in a natural environment' (p.173). It was considered to be important to structure the environment like this because of the challenge presented by the 'outside' world to a construct system which is too loose and unstructured.

Even so it was not possible to achieve the kind of control over the environment which would have made the task of identifying and validating specific constructs really practicable. There was too much 'noise' in the system to identify any clear signal which could be amplified without distortion, although this seems to have had more to do with distracting social interaction outside the experimental environment than breakdown of relationship within: 'the experimental intervention represented a single theme in the patient's life which was continually being contradicted and confused by other themes' (1975: 178).

At the same time, the investigators came across a more important problem in trying to communicate with patients, one which was not entirely due to looseness of constructs, although it was clearly connected with this. This was the special use of language in which disordered thinking was compounded by idiosyncratic meanings ascribed to the words used. In other words the private languages employed were not simply inefficient forms of public communication, but diverged from normality at a more basic semantic level than expected. Content, as well as structure had been affected. A different approach seemed to be demanded, one avoiding the impression of 'scientists' conducting an 'experiment' on passive subjects. Bannister suggests that in order to achieve the quality of communication necessary to validate patient's constructs the approach should come from the patients themselves, who should be encouraged to create settings in which the kind of relationship they need in order to feel accepted ('validated') in their own ways of interpreting the world can be fostered: 'It might be seen as a matter of allowing ourselves to be used by the patient so that he can validate himself (e.g. as someone able to form interpersonal relationships). Future work on the idea might well start from the premise that patients must be allowed to create their own worlds in which they can explore relationship with each other and the therapist.'

Drama therapy aims at helping individuals create worlds that can be shared. This is an ambitious project in the case of those in whom 'social communication is crowded out by fantasy' (Cameron, 1944: 51). Nevertheless it must be undertaken if we are to help people whose sense of self-with-regard-to-others is poorly developed. The kind of interchange of being which we have recognised as the essence of personhood only takes place from a secure centre. On the other hand, security and stability are themselves functions of the process of interaction. As Kelly says 'to the extent that one person construes the construction processes of another, they may play a role in a social process involving another person' (1955: 95). Interaction is itself necessary to establish the personal reality of those engaged in it. Psychology reiterates what dramatic theory has always understood: to be fully human we must possess the ability to experience reality in and through others. Just as Goffman regards society as dramaturgically constructed, an artistic attempt at social communication carried on by means of the self-conscious 'presentation' of selected aspects of an over-all inter-personal reality (1971), so Kelly describes a similar process occurring at a micro-social level, in which individuals 'try out for size' various views of themselves as perceived by other people, so as to select the ones which allow them to carry on social relationships with one another. Kelly sees our personal role as continually changing, as we adjust and readjust our own personal picture of the relationship we want to establish or maintain. This is something very like Jung's 'active imagination', active not only for art but for life as well.

The fact that artistic theory can be used to explain personal breakdown itself suggests an artistic approach to therapy, one which attempts by artistic means to help disorientated people achieve greater psychological stability. As we have seen, if our sense of self has been rarely, or only intermittently, validated we will tend to play safe, be unwilling to take chances in our dealings with other people, either by remaining in an entrenched position or refusing to allow ourselves to be tied down at all, states of mind associated by Bannister and Fransella with obsessionality and schizophrenia (1986: 77). The process of validation must involve not simply the provision of an environment which is emotionally secure, as is the case with depression, but one which is structurally recognisable, in which role relationships are clearly defined and different kinds of human experience, laughter,sadness, work, play, formality and informality, are taken in context, each, and each combination of each, receiving validation from recognisable authorities in circumstances widely regarded as being appropriate. In ordinary social life, commu-nication largely depends on the order in which events take place. Human meaning is circumstantial in that it is when – and, of course, where – we choose to say and do things that transmits our message. As Goffman points out, the processes whereby this shaping is carried out are frequently overlooked or actually concealed. In the drama these same stratagems of human role playing are clearly revealed. The 'validational schedules' of personal relationship stand clearly revealed and may be studied: if we are taking part ourselves, they may be safely practised. In Construct Theory terms, the process of loosening and tightening is considerably less frightening than in life, because the range of events to be anticipated is drastically limited, and our involvement in them entirely voluntary.

Here, at last, is a form of personal experience we can focus upon with confidence because we can afford to get it wrong. To this extent drama is both a play ground for the release of inter-personal tension and a laboratory for the safe anticipation of events. Even more importantly, it is the clarification of the structures which validate our experience of life. Certainly, because of difficulties concerning the boundaries of the sense of self, what Stanislavski characterises as the 'as if' faculty in human perception seems curiously lacking in schizophrenic people (1936: 43–49). This in itself would suggest that drama is likely to present very real difficulties for them because of an inability to see the other without homogenisation or alienation as *someone else who might be me.* If I am unable to say 'this is different from that, yet both are significant or meaningful from different points of view or with reference to different criteria of truthfulness' I am unable to move freely among alternative ways of interpreting the world that confronts and contains me. I am unable to make use of one viewpoint as a way of explaining, or expanding, another, and my 'epistemological repertoire' is too limited, and consequently too inflexible, for the kind of cross-referencing other people take for granted.[7]

Drama consists specifically in acting as if I were someone else and knowing that I am doing so. For this reason it is particularly relevant to the kind of thought disorder associated with schizophrenia. Like drama itself, it is an arrangement of forms – roles, conventions, contrasts, similarities, modes of understanding, images and feelings – which encourages us to discriminate between a range of different ways, and kinds of ways, of perceiving. Nothing is haphazard; all are closely related, either by similarity or difference, to one another. Where there is confusion, this too is distinguished: it is confusion *as opposed to* order. Structure is employed in a conscious or intentional way, in order to reveal its true identity as the means by which we relate things in order to make sense of them. In this way, Drama therapy helps perception to achieve a particular kind of clarity, providing it with the raw material for involvement with a world in which contrasts are heightened and similarities underlined. It is its power to reveal the structure of common reality which makes it valuable for schizophrenics, who suffer from a chronic inability to recognise important structural distinctions in the reality which involves and confronts them, and for whom structure is often invented rather than received. As a result, there is often no clearly discernible relationship between the thought-world of the individual and that of his or her neighbours. The schizophrenic person is unable to distinguish clearly what is going on around him or her, to discriminate between what is, what might be, and what definitely is not happening, and so draws private conclusions which do not always fit the public facts.

We have seen how this confusion may have originated, as an individual's attempts to draw conclusions about the state of affairs existing with regard to his or her relationships with other people are systematically invalidated by the chronic presence of conflicting evidence. Whether this state of affairs is the negative result of an organic condition, or represents a positive attempt to cope with the demands of an insupportable inter-personal situation which they have contrived for themselves (Sullivan, 1974), such people need clarity in their perception of others. There is evidence that experience of drama can be particularly therapeutic.

Up to now we have been mainly concerned with explanations of the healing power of drama. In Part II we shall consider a particular example of this power. Before that, however, it might be helpful once again to identify the effects of the dramatic experience that make it an unique healing force.

(1) *katharsis* through engulfment or psychological involvement evoked by the action of the play's structure on the imagination of those concerned. The result is an intensification of the conditions of human relationship which is experienced as emotionally healing because it increases our courage to be ('validates' us), and persuades us of the viability of alternative ways of being ('as if').

(2) *psychological integration* through the provision of a vital link between 'inner' and 'outer' reality. Relationship with other people depends on our relationship with our own fantasy life in which the symbolism of communication with others originates. We learn to take account of the independent reality of other people by identifying objects, images and, later on, ideas, which can be developed into ways of sharing experience and understanding. Our first experience of art is interior, although its specific form may relate to an awareness of the power of art to communicate truth of a pre-verbal kind. The integration of the alienated psyche is promoted by constructing an imaginative bridge with the outside world.

(3) *security* for people who fear engulfment by others and so 'close in on themselves', construing their personal worlds tightly in order not to leave themselves open to danger. By manipulating aesthetic distance drama fosters a sense of personal boundaries which permits genuine relationship. This is particularly helpful for depressed people who construe the world tightly for defensive purposes. It is not at odds with (a), as drama consists in an oscillation of engulfment and separation – that is, it is itself an image of the way we construe our personal reality. Being involved with and standing back from other people we build up a picture of the reality which contains us and them. Drama addresses itself to the loneliness of depression and is taken up eagerly by people who have much to express, but little sense of their own value. This leads on to –

(4) *validation*, attempts at making sense of an experience of life which is essentially nonsensical, arbitrary, self-contradictory, confusing. We need to be able to discern a degree of regularity in the things that happen to us before we can organise them into any kind of pattern and create the kind of behavioural and cognitive map in which past, present and future can be used to explain one another. Generally speaking, drama makes better sense of showing how things fit together than life does, because it drastically limits the elements to be construed while extending the time available for construing them before the flux of events can alter their meaning. For this reason it is of help to people whose thought is disordered.

Notes

1. 'The focus of schizophrenic confusion' (may be located as) '"thinking about people" rather than "thinking about things"'. – D. Bannister, F. Salmon (1966: 219).

2. Bateson and his fellow workers describe four factors which contribute to the situation in its classical form: 1) *Dramatis personae*, indicating a 'victim' and an individual or group which inflicts harm on him. (This may be the mother or father alone, or a combination of parents and siblings). 2) *Mise en scène*. The double-bind is not a single traumatic experience, but a habitual expectation – part of the environment in fact. 3) *Negative directions* – 'Do not do so-and-so, or I punish you', or 'If you do not do so-and-so, I will punish you' – plus: 4) *Conflicting directions*. These cut across the original directions at a higher level of abstraction. Both injunctions are enforced by the threat of punishment or the withdrawal of a sustaining relationship perceived by the victim as vital for his safety or even survival.

3. For example, a 'skewed' family in which one parent is totally dominated by the other broadcasts itself as ideally balanced; a close, warm relationship is claimed in a marriage where one parent's coldness and emotional withdrawal has caused a 'schism' to form between them. Either of these distorted views of reality, says Lidz, may be imposed upon the child by parents 'whose emotional equilibrium is so tenuous that (they) can maintain (their) stability only by perceiving events according to (their) needs and by insisting that others distort their perceptions as (they) do' (1975: 33).

4. Perhaps this adds to the 'flatness of affect' characterising schizophrenic behaviour.

5. 'The schizophrenic thought disorder is a complex resultant of the parents' amorphous or fragmented styles of communicating, of poor training in categorising, of having been taught paranoid mistrust within the home, of the paralogical thinking that results from trying to elude the double-bind, of thinking irrationally to suit the parents' egocentric needs, and intrusions of vague inter-categorical polymorphous infantile and early childhood fantasies. The therapist,' Lidz continues, 'can counter the patient's over-inclusive thinking and enhance focal attention by fostering clear boundaries between the patient and others, particularly between the patient and the therapist, by being consistent and clear in his communications...' (1975: 113, 114).

6. For example, in 1975, Bannister, Adams-Webber, Penn and Radley attempted 'to reverse the process of thought-disorder by first identifying whatever weak, remaining system of expectations the thought-disordered patient manifests and then fulfilling these expectations.' It was hypothesised that 'such a process of serial validation might lead to a strengthening of the 'theory' which generated these

expectations – a tightening of the construct system.' The results showed a treatment effect which was statistically non-significant (1975).

7. The 'concrete thinking' associated with schizophrenia has no use for the metaphors which enrich normal perception. How can it have, when it cannot see beyond itself and its own immediate reality? In the same way, the absence of distance between self and other, the confusion which at the same time is a crippling restriction, obviates the need for real personal communication. Why should I struggle to make things clear when I know exactly what I mean? Hence, because the argument is familiar to the person propounding it, stages vital to the other person are omitted: the celebrated 'knight's move' of schizophrenic symptomatology.

Part II

Process

Chapter 5

Approaches to Drama Therapy

Up to now I have concentrated on establishing the relationship of drama to healing processes. From this point I shall adopt a more practical position and refer to ways in which the therapeutic power of drama can be harnessed. Whereas Part I has been largely concerned with theory, Part II will move into more personal areas, dealing with people as well as ideas, and finding them considerably harder to pin down. Much of the healing effect of drama depends on the freedom and spontaneity with which we respond to one another. In practical terms of living in the world of real men and women, freedom and spontaneity take a good deal of arranging.

In this chapter some of the vital structural elements which underlie and support the dramatherapeutic process are briefly described. None of them happen automatically: all need painstaking preparation and a lot of careful thought. How, for instance, can people be encouraged to feel both secure and challenged, relaxed and yet alert? It is this vital element of structure that provides the key to the healing work of drama. Because of its combination of *structure* (character, plot and presentation) and *freedom* (from the demands of extra-dramatic reality) drama is experienced as liberating by those who find themselves oppressed by a narrow and restrictive sense of themselves as an independent person, as in depressed states, or by their lack of any stable and recognisable image of the self, as in schizoid conditions. Therapeutic approaches based on drama are able to provide easily identifiable models of personal interaction and to be both safe and challenging at the same time. Dramatic structure has been shown to provide people suffering from disordered thinking with the kind of experience of human interaction which they can use to give shape to their own lives.[1] It speaks the language of human intentions and emotions instead of merely using language to speak about them. The kind of drama which provides the medium for drama therapy is the basic material of everyday experience, the kind of dialogue which springs unbidden to our lips.

Most important of all, the therapist's central task, is the setting of the scene – the largely invisible structure which will provide a milieu for the exploration of ideas and experience, moving us away from things that are well-established and familiar into the world of imaginative possibility. To do this, certain ground rules have to be established. Establishing or creating an atmosphere of mutual acceptance and regard is necessary for the unique combination of safety and danger which makes drama therapy such an effective way of treating people who are ontologically vulnerable. Advances in self-identification are rooted in the experience of self-acceptance which proceeds from the validation of things as they are. For example, if I am to relinquish a particular restrictive or self-punitive attitude to myself, I must be given specific permission to let go of it. This must be done as explicitly as possible, as it is in the following exchange, which takes place in a group of eight people:

Leader: How are you feeling today, Joan?

Joan: I feel nervous. *(She is clutching a cushion, and obviously wishes she hadn't joined the group today)*

Leader: I can see. You're holding the cushion very tightly, aren't you?

Joan: I'll put it down. *(She doesn't)*

Leader: What shall we do with it?

Betty: I'll take it off her. *(She goes across to Joan, smiles at her and relieves her of the cushion)*

John: Now you've got it. What are you going to do with it?

Betty: What shall I do with it? *(There is a pause in which everybody looks at the Leader, who says nothing. Eventually Joan speaks)*

Joan: Chuck it away.

Betty: Shall I?

Joan: Yes. Chuck it away. We don't need a cushion, do we?

(Philip, another member of the group, takes the cushion and throws it into a corner of the room, well outside the circle)

In this way, everybody present takes advantages of the 'special circumstances' of the group to share as many people's attitudes as they can, drawing spiritual strength from the fact that the group itself has its own corporate identity which is at every member's disposal.

(1) Roles

Much of what is done in a session of drama therapy, both in the games played, with their fixed rules, and in the improvised exploration of dramatic episodes, is based upon the notion of role-reversal. This embodies another basic principle, that of mutual concern.

> *(Andrew mentions that he has had an argument with the man next door about the noise of his record player. He is obviously upset about this, and wants to talk about it to the group. He is still too angry to be very coherent, however.)*

Andrew: I can't tell you what it was like. He said…

Leader: Perhaps you can show us. Would somebody like to be Andrew's neighbour? *(Pause, while everybody considers what to do. Jim goes over to Andrew and stands in front of him, taking up an aggressive posture)*

Jim: Oh, it's you, is it?

Andrew: Get lost. *(We are not sure whether this is addressed to Jim personally, or in his role as neighbour).*

Jim: What's the matter? You usually make enough noise in all conscience! *(This gets through to Andrew, who proceeds to mount a verbal attack on the neighbour, seeming to have forgotten it is Jim that he's 'really' talking to).*

After a few minutes, roles are reversed; Andrew plays the neighbour and Jim takes over as Andrew. Other members of the group join in, so that there are eventually several Andrews, each putting his point of view about the record player, and several neighbours determined to hold their own on the subject of noise abatement. In this way customary modes of self-presentation are loosened by imaginative participation in the shared emotional life of the group.[2]

In drama therapy one is required to take account of several different kinds of relationship, all based upon the fundamental mechanism of role reversal and requiring a range of mental operations which are separate and yet confusingly similar, all taking place within the same event. Johnson analyses the process as follows:

'A. *Impersonal:* the relationship between two enacted roles (e.g. 'Bob-as-salesman' and 'Jane-as-customer')

B. *Intrapersonal:* the relationship between each person and his own role (e.g. Bob and the 'salesman' and Jane and the 'customer')

C. *Extrapersonal:* the relationship between each person and the other person's role, (e.g. Bob and the 'customer' and Jane and the 'salesman')

D. *Interpersonal:* the relationship between the two individuals (e.g. Bob and Jane)' (1981B: 53)

The last of these, the interpersonal, is emotionally the most highly charged. Indeed, the achievement of a higher level of spontaneity and engagement in this area is the object of the exercise. The four levels are closely connected, however, because security in inter-personal relationship governs the making of relational distinctions in general. From another point of view, the intrapersonal is crucial. If a clear line of demarcation can be established at this level, between the self as it experiences itself, and as it has contrived to present itself (i.e. as 'someone else'), a degree of *solidity* has been bestowed upon the 'real' self which may be put to good use at the level of the interpersonal. I am no longer transparent in my dealings with other people, because I have two distinct ways of being towards them. I can 'be myself', or I can 'play a role'. This primary division of function is explored in its variations at the levels of the impersonal and the extrapersonal, so that the complete exercise may provide a kind of lived-through illustration of the basic range of options available to the individual self in performing its primary function of boundary manipulation for purposes of contact with, and preservation from, other people. Once this paradigm has been assimilated, reality may be less threatening simply because it is more understandable. It is more understandable here because it is not presented as an interesting idea, but as something that is actually lived through. By participating in the exercise, we demonstrate to ourselves the reality of the experience it involves us in. Things which may be hard to grasp by thinking about are fleshed out in the doing.

(2) Games

Rule two calls for the acceptance of the therapeutic value of games, used as a way of helping people to relax, both physically and psychologically. The fact that it is a game is the sole justification for an event, not simply an excuse offered to patients for something they might find embarrassing, or a way of distracting their attention from its therapeutic purpose. Thus, people are given permission to enjoy themselves and helped to lose their self-consciousness. Once a group of people have become attuned to one another through the experience of imaginative play, all kinds of adjustments can be made in the way they are able to allow themselves to perceive themselves, their companions and the world in general. It is as if a process of group adjustment takes place within the special protected world of the game, a kind of corporate homeostatic movement in which each individual finds a kind of balance through inviting the others into his or her own universe. In this place, at this time, we receive permission to be ourselves and encouragement to explore the possibilities of new kinds of selfhood that are revealed to us. As Smail says: 'it is often helpful to encourage patients to *trust* their non-reflective unselfconscious activity, since the ultimate aim of psychotherapy can only be to enable the person to set off down paths he does not already know' (1978: 110).

This kind of game-playing approach underlies all drama therapy. It is particularly appropriate to the treatment of anxiety states. The following example is from Dorothy Langley (1983) and represents Session 2 in a three session programme for people suffering from social anxiety:

'(1) Group forms a circle, A goes into the middle and starts miming an action, B joins him but by his action shows that he feels of higher status than A. C now enters the circle and shows he is of a higher status than B. A leaves the circle. Either continue raising the status or lowering it alternatively until the group have all had a turn.

(2) In pairs A is master and B is servant and has to obey every command without question. Reverse roles.

(3) Repeat, but this time the servant gradually becomes higher in status until he becomes the master.

(4) Discuss what you have done so far. What status do people prefer? Discuss situations which called for altered status. How do we behave towards our bank manager and the attendant of the petrol pump?

(5) In pairs, A wants to enter a road but B tries to prevent him verbally. Look at the roles people select for themselves – policeman, gas board inspector etc. Compare the status each has selected. Then ask the group to repeat the scene but reversing status (not roles) e.g. if A is a low-status delivery man and B is a high status policeman, then A becomes a high status delivery man and B a low status policeman. (This is a difficult exercise and groups may feel unable to cope with it. The point is to identify the kind of speech and body language that reflects high/low status. There should be plenty of opportunity to discuss this as it is basic to the rest of the course. If necessary, let it take until the end of the session).

(6) Divide into small groups. The scene is a station waiting room: each person chooses a role and enters the improvisation when he is ready. As each new character appears the others react to the status he portrays.' (Langley, 1983: 129–130)

Some of the games played in the course of programmes of drama therapy require a much greater degree of flexibility in the way in which we see ourselves than we normally achieve. The discovery that we can in fact amuse ourselves in ways that are so very different from the habitual behaviour of our public selves can be an important stage in learning about ourselves. As people start to feel stronger and more at peace with themselves and the world, they complain less about being made to feel childish and conspicuous when they are asked to do something 'just for fun'.

(3) Sculpts

To make personal communication as clear as possible bodily gestures and positions are used to express states of mind. This takes practice, because we are all used to expressing ourselves verbally, to the exclusion of any of the other ways at our disposal. Bodily positions are unequivocal, even when the intention is to express mixed feelings. The physical disposition of bodies, the degree of closeness to and distance from others presents the reality of personal and social relationship in ways that escape language. Words may be used, of course, but the primary mode of self-expression remains physical, as in the technique known as 'sculpting', in which a person or group create a statue to symbolise a particular idea or experience, some acting as sculptors, the rest as clay, before reversing the process to play one another's roles. The symbolic power of movement and posture provides drama therapy with a useful shorthand for summarising complex relationships. Just as importantly, however, it encourages those taking part to become more aware of, and take personal responsibility for, their bodies, which provide the essential physical evidence of their presence in the real world of men and women. Bodies interact, they do not merge. There is as much to be learnt about identity and consequently about relationship, from bodies as there is from minds. Dramatherapy employs the physical presence of men and women in order to structure experiences of separation and engulfment.

(4) Metaphor

Without metaphor drama cannot exist. This is in some ways the most fundamental rule of all. Metaphor is to be nurtured as a means to self-expression and self-discovery. Drama itself is a metaphorical activity, a way of presenting life 'at one remove'. In drama therapy much of the subject matter, as well as the artistic form, is metaphorical. The stories used have a symbolic resonance which may relate to what is perceived to be the meaning of life by those taking part. Scenarios taken from legend, folk-lore and mythology recur frequently in work generated by the group, not only in that supplied in advance by the leader. A fairy-tale or even a nursery rhyme can unlock a world of imaginative creativity which goes undiscovered when group members remain determinedly earth-bound. It is important that they return to earth again, but when they do they are likely to say they feel differently because of the experience, which has put them in touch with things about themselves that had remained unacknowledged and unexpressed. The ability of meta-phor to remind people of ideas and feelings not present in their conscious awareness gives rise to a powerful reaction in those sensitive to any invasion of areas of the self which are too painful to be disturbed; on the other hand the metaphor itself provides a measure of safety, as our reasoning intellect reassures that it is 'only a play'. For safety reasons, it is advisable to talk about what has happened on the journey the group has been engaged in, as this allays some of the disturbance. The journey itself remains a real experience to be both remembered and benefited from. Metaphors which involve a perilous journey in which a mountain must be climbed, an ocean crossed, or a cave or forest penetrated, embody the individual's release from anxiety as the group arrive triumphantly at their destination, having endured and triumphed.

Journeys of a mythic kind involving the use of symbols of psychic transformation require very careful work to set the scene. The action may involve movement and speech and take all the available space for its terrain or it may take place entirely in the imagination of group members who, without leaving their chairs, follow wherever they are led. Either way it should begin with a series of exercises in relaxation. If it is to be an imaginary journey those taking part are first of all instructed to close their eyes in order to concentrate on what is happening: when everybody is sitting or lying down, in the most comfortable position they can find, the Leader begins to speak. Quietly, in a voice which is contrived to be both soothing and expressive, the Leader describes a journey that everyone is taking, out of the familiar surroundings of the room into whatever lies beyond. Although the whole group is involved, each person journeys alone. 'You are walking along a road. It is night. On each side of you mountains loom away to the sky. You can hardly see the sky, though, because the mountains are so steep and tall. What can you see? How do you feel? You kick your boots through the sand of the trail... This is where the trail forks. One path leads on down the valley, and the other twists up into the mountain.' The Leader explains that the path leads upwards to the home of 'a very Wise Person who can tell the answer to any question.' The trail is followed, and the Wise Person discovered, sitting in front of a cave on the mountainside. Each group member asks what he or she most wishes to know, and receives, not a verbal reply, but an object of some kind to take back down the mountain. Everybody says goodbye to the Wise Person and they all return down the mountain, along the trail, and thence into the room where they are sitting or lying. They open their eyes.

Obviously a session like this requires a good deal of concentration on the part of group members and some skill in story-telling on the part of the Leader, who must present the material as evocatively as possible. The image of the Wise Person is an immensely powerful one (as Jung discovered). The job of the Leader is to let it speak for itself. It is possible to explore the idea further by encouraging people to exchange roles with the Wise Person and so, metaphorically, to take on the wisdom he/she epitomises. Whether or not this happens, it is essential that the gifts he/she has bestowed are presented by each person in turn to the group, either verbally, by describing them, or pictorially, with the help of actions, drawings or models.

Different people find difficulty in different things. Much of the skill of the Leader of a drama therapy session lies in gauging the degree of challenge represented by various processes, so that group members are stimulated rather than discouraged. This is easier when dealing with a group sharing the same problem, than with one where there are some members who are depressed, some confused, others anxious or obsessional. Can the same material help everyone? In fact, the outcome may be favourable when clients interact to give one another encouragement and support. In every case, however, it is vitally important to begin at the lowest achievable level of threat – in other words to start very simply at the level of getting to know one another. The following is a brief description of a course of drama therapy consisting of 10 one-hour sessions designed for a group of patients at a psychiatric day hospital. Here there were ten members, including the Leader. Two of the patients had been referred because they suffered from anxiety; three were considered to be thought-disordered and one, at least, was depressed. Because of the range of conditions represented the programme dealt with various aspects of interpersonal activity, starting with simple exercises fostering awareness of others, and becoming progressively more complex and demanding as it required a greater ability to predict other people's behaviour and to share their feelings. The areas covered were:

Session 1   Awareness of another's physical presence.

Session 2   Sharing information about one's self with someone else.

Session 3   Trusting another person in a make-believe (dramatic) situation.

Session 4   Sharing tasks with another person in real-life situations.

Session 5   Sharing tasks within the group.

Session 6   Relationship as self-expression. (Expressing the self in terms of awareness of others)

Session 7   Creating a 'world' (i.e. a consistently organised social situation) via the imagination and sharing it with the group.

Session 8   Exploring alternative ways of presenting the self.

Session 9   Self disclosure 'at one remove' (i.e. using a metaphor or symbol)

Session 10   Disclosing the ways in which one's personal world is structured.

All sessions involved 'putting oneself in another's place'. The difference between sessions 1, 6 and 10 can be clearly seen.

Session 1

The Leader invites everyone to sit in a circle. He/she introduces himself. The purpose of these 10 sessions is to help people get to know one another and enjoy knowing one another better. People don't have to stay if they don't want to. If they want to come back and join in again, they may. Any questions?

Group Exchange names, members introducing themselves *ad lib.*, with help of Leader. People find partners.

Pairs 'Mirroring' – 'A' moves a part of his/her body, say a hand, very slowly. 'B' follows each movement as closely as possible. The hands are held very close to each other. ('See if you can feel the heat from the other person's hand!') With some practice you can move slowly enough to deceive a spectator as to who is leading. After a minute or so, when the Leader calls 'change', 'A' and 'B' exchange roles. This can be varied.

One partner turns his/her back while the other makes a slight adjustment in his/her appearance, then asks partner to say what has been changed. This is repeated in reverse order.

Pairs spend a few minutes exchanging views on a subject of topical interest suggested by Leader.

Group Each member reports his/her partner's comments on the topic (having gained partner's permission). He does this by pretending to be his partner – 'I am…, and I said…etc.'

Group Members are encouraged to group one another according to a shared characteristic. People stand together in their groups.

Goodbye – shake hands or hug.

Session 6

Group *(seated in circle)* Names game – each member says his/her name and throws bean-bag to someone else, who says his/her name, and so on.

Group *(standing in circle)* What did we do last week? How did you feel about it? (Contributions invited)

Greet someone in a way intended to make them feel better. Choose partners.

Partners You are a sculptor and your partner is a lump of clay. Make a sculpture of him/her in a pose which is characteristic of him/her. Walk round and inspect the other 'sculpts'. Wind your own 'sculpt' up and set him/her 'going' (i.e. like a robot).

Now put him/her in an uncharacteristic pose, and repeat the procedure of inspection and animation. Change places with your partner and repeat as above.

Groups   Each group chooses a feeling or an emotion and does a 'group sculpt' in which all the group members put themselves and one another into poses expressive of the emotion. (The result should look like a complicated piece of statuary). Having done this, they transfer to an emotion which is directly opposite to the one they started with (e.g. anxiety-calmness, or vice versa). Groups show each other their sculpts and try to guess the feelings portrayed.

Group   (seated) Each member writes down the name of a feeling or an emotion on a piece of paper. These are shuffled, and everyone takes a new piece. What sort of thing makes you feel the emotion written on the paper you have drawn from the pile? Each member talks about each emotion.

Quiet goodbyes.

Session 10

Group   (standing) Members stand in a circle clasping hands. One member tightens his grip with one of his hands. Receiving this, his neighbour tightens his own grip on *his* neighbour's hand and the pressure is passed round the circle. Still holding hands, the group sways gently to the right, then to the left, while members say hello to one another. People get chairs and sit in a circle.

Group   (seated) Members say what the week has been like for them. (This can be mimed or sculpted).

Leader   places a chair in the ring, and asks each member to place an article – a book, a lighter, a key – on or near the chair. What has been happening here? Can you invent a scene which would explain why these objects are here? The group divides into two in order to devise similar scenarios, and test each other's skill in guessing them. This is discussed, and may lead into the subject of the kind of things that happen in families...

Group   Someone in the group volunteers to 'cast' people in the role of members of his/her family. These people are grouped together in accordance with the person's feelings about how 'close' (emotionally involved with) they are to one another and to him/her. Having done this he/she moves round the group he/she has created and speaks in character as each family member (e.g. if Phyllis were depicting her family like this, she might go up to Tom, whom she had chosen to represent her father and put her hand on his shoulder and say 'I am Fred, Phyllis's Dad, and I think... I feel...) Next, each member of the family group speaks up as if they were the people they have been asked to represent, using the information given them about their characters in the previous stage of the exercise, and supplementing this with their own insights concerning Phyllis's family.

It is unlikely that there will be enough time to do this for more than one or two people present. However, this is an exercise which involves everybody within the atmosphere of empathy and self-disclosure it sets out to create. Some time should be left at the end of the session for discussion and 'de-roleing'. As this is the final session in this programme, group members must have time and encouragement to review their experiences during the last 10 weeks. Having reached this point, they should have the opportunity to proceed further.

This was an introductory course of sessions. It is not always necessary to plan things out like this. Indeed it may be counter-productive, as the most exciting developments occur spontaneously. So long as the basic principles of freedom-in-structure are borne in mind a therapist may trust his or her instincts about the subject matter, picking up impressions from the group and developing them dramatically, and encouraging individual members to do the same. What is important, however, is the way that things are brought to a close at the end of a session. This seems obvious, but because of the interest and excitement aroused by whatever has been going on, the closing stage is often neglected. At its worst, this can mean that group members cannot easily adjust to the return to normality. Having spent half-an-hour 'in role' as somebody entirely different from themselves, it can be disturbing to have to relinquish their new-found identity so brusquely. It is even more confusing if nothing is said or done at all, and they have to leave the session not knowing who they are supposed to be. Some way – a short game perhaps – must be found of confirming them as themselves.

Notes

1. Grainger (1987).
2. The notion of role reversal is fundamental to the thinking of Jakob Moreno, founder of psychodrama. His clinical work with individual patients led him to regard the action of agreeing to exchange identity with another person as one of the most psychologically invigorating actions of which human beings are capable. Indeed, it was the key to the kind of spontaneous experience of emotional katharsis which

greatly reduces a troubled individual's preoccupation with his or her own personal private universe of thoughts and feelings. 'Reversing of roles with all the individuals and objects of one's social universe seems to be, at least theoretically, an indispensable requirement for the establishment of a psychodramatic community' (1972: 142). Where role reversal is too difficult, because a person's sense of identity is insufficiently strong, 'doubling' techniques might be used instead:— 'A lonely child, like a schizophrenic patient, may never be able to do a role reversal but he will accept a double: that is, somebody who will assume his identity and speak up on his behalf' (1972: 157). However, the crucial technique of role reversal is not something which has to be imposed, because it comes quite naturally to human beings. Indeed children find it exceedingly easy to do, and benefit from practising the technique. Moreno's experiments in psychodramatic play with his own son Jonathan led him to state that 'role reversal increases the strength and stability of the child's ego: ego is here defined as identity with himself.' The principle seems to be quite straightforward: the more confident I become at playing your role, the surer I am of my own! In order to play you I must be doubly sure of myself. In particular, the ideas, attitudes and feelings which distinguish me from you must be fully recognised and acknowledged before they can be temporarily suspended. This is something I do not need to be taught, although I may need reminding of it.

Chapter 6

Some of the Cast

It is as necessary in drama therapy as in other forms of therapy to take case-histories so as to arrive at some kind of overall view of an individual person's life, feelings, ideas and objectives. The four histories presented in this chapter depend largely on techniques of self-reportage, adopting what Kelly calls the 'credulous approach'. This is a method which tries to take account of what is actually said by the person concerned, keeping hermeneutic intervention to a minimum. The individual reveals him or herself in whatever is disclosed or held back, and whatever emerges from the dramatherapeutic process itself in the form of definite communication. Obviously, it is impossible to eliminate the element of interpretation altogether, but the aim is always to preserve the individual's intended meaning rather than the therapist's pre-conceived construction of its significance. Sometimes self-disclosure is more revealing when it happens unawares or is mediated by someone else; this is why notes on the sessions have been included. To begin with we did not 'present' the histories or episodes contained in them in psychodramatic form. By giving their histories in this way, people located themselves and others in a narrative plot which had its own dramatic power in the telling, giving meaning and shape, and setting the scene for drama in the sessions to come.

TM – Age 57

T was born in Lincolnshire, the only son of parents who lived in a small village, several miles from the nearest town. He says that his childhood was 'happy enough – you knew where you stood in a place like that.' When pressed on this point, he went on to say that he had appreciated 'knowing his place' in a 'proper community.' This being the case it is not perhaps surprising that when he was old enough to do so, T joined the police force. He married at nineteen, a local girl, and soon afterwards they moved to live in a small urban village near Wakefield. This first marriage did not last very long. T is not forthcoming about the reasons for its breaking down, but he soon married again. T's new wife came to him with two sons, and having no children by his first wife, T tried hard to make a new start in unfamiliar conditions: 'I tried to build a new life by running the household in an ordered way.' Unfortunately this was an up-hill struggle. T complains that his new wife never contributed by making any effort to keep things in order, leaving it all to him. Sixteen months before T came to the Day Hospital he moved out 'in despair.' Since then, he has been 'courting her again, hoping to get her to change her ways.' How unsuccessful the attempt had been was revealed by the fact that his wife had just shattered all his hopes in the most dramatic way: 'She has made a confession of adultery and we've filed for divorce.' T dwelt for a long time on the details of his narrative concerning his discovery of her 'betrayal'. He was also very conscious of his own isolation, and complained that he could get no support or understanding from his wife's parents who, he felt, had colluded with her in encouraging her to cohabit with her lover in the marital home, an arrangement which T found deeply shocking.

T looks exceptionally fit, and is always smartly dressed, in a rather 'dashing' fashion. The cottage he lives in is scrupulously neat and tidy, and this may be taken to be characteristic of T's attitude to life. He prefers places to be neat and tidy and situations to be clear and unambiguous. For example, it was noticed at the Day Hospital that he tended to take TV dramas very seriously, as if he recognised no difference between 'ordinary life' and drama, regarding plays as documentary programmes, and that he had difficulty in gauging people's responses in conversation with them — both signs of an unsubtle, inflexible way of construing inter-personal situations. He is uneasy with metaphors, tending to take things literally. (At the same time, however, he enjoys painting, and when I went to see him at home I noticed a row of small pictures he had done, arranged along the edge of the bed and propped up against the wall. The pictures were all factual representations, sea-scapes and country scenes, all neatly set out in a row, as tidy as T himself.)

The Day Hospital staff noticed from the beginning that T was very rank-conscious. He asked each nurse their designation and place within the hierarchy and tried hard to distinguish himself from the other patients, sitting at the far end of the room, as if he were trying to reassure himself that reliable social divisions existed within the new world of the Day Hospital, as they did, or were supposed to do, outside. A sense of order and purpose in life that was probably not very well-developed to begin with, and needed to be constantly reaffirmed, had been severely impaired by recent events. T wept when he spoke about his wife, but they were tears of frustration, not love: his carefully restored pattern had been vandalised, and he could do nothing to put the pieces back together again. He was hard to talk to on the subject, because he would take nothing 'on trust', demanding that everything be explained to him. On the other hand, 'talking about things' is believed to be the only solution to the problem; if people talk long enough everything is bound to fall into place, and life will be controllable once more.

While he was at the Day Hospital, T found out that his wife and her lover were receiving separate social security benefits despite the fact that they were living together. T was determined to put an end to this by informing the authorities. Any sense of personal loyalty that remained was rendered inoperative by his determination to uphold the Law.

T joined in most of the exercises in the drama therapy programme, but made it quite clear that he did not see the point of them. He had no objection to joining a group, but preferred to run things himself. In the Bannister and Fransella Thought Disorder Test he found it difficult to arrange photographs into different categories according to the characteristic portrayed by the people represented. Once he had made his original choices he found it hard to change his viewpoint (e.g. when he had ranked the photographs in order of varying degrees of 'kindness', for example, he baulked at the idea of rearranging them in varying degrees of 'stupidity': 'I've ordered them once, I can't change them round to fit something else'). On analysis, T's grids reveal a tendency to employ a few basic constructs which are kept comparatively isolated from one another. Things – and people – are filed into separate compartments, and the key to the cabinet is held firmly by T. In Construct Theory terms, his construing is overly pre-emptive and this is as limiting as a loose and ill-defined system when it comes to efficiency in predicting and controlling events. If people can only act in one way, only be one kind of person, what happens when they don't? You might as well suspend your judgement about them altogether.

Sessions 1–3. T obviously thought the sessions childish, and said so, whenever the group was invited to pass comments about what they were thinking and feeling. He enjoyed taking the initiative in those exercises which he did not consider too infantile. The 'guided fantasy' in Session 2 was tolerated, but not enjoyed: 'It didn't do anything for *me*!' The finger painting, however, was much better received, as T is talented in this direction, and his unwillingness to abandon 'proper' brushes and 'scrabble about like a baby' was outweighed by the opportunity to display his artistic skills.

Sessions 4–5. T was unwilling – or unable – to abandon his dignity long enough to contribute much to the dramatic improvisations in Sessions IV and V, and amused himself by 'sending things up'. As a respecter of authority, he never did this openly, preferring to make one or two of the other people present laugh behind the leader's back. In other words he avoided feeling childish by behaving like a child. Usually he was trying to attract the attention of one of the women in the group to whom he was attracted. (On one of the Day Hospital questionnaires, T noted that he 'no longer had any sexual feelings', so this may have been vanity.) This situation, in which T played out his own 'private' drama against the background of the main activity of the session, was to continue for the rest of the programme, to the exasperation of almost everybody except the two people concerned.

Sessions 6–7. By this stage in the programme T was beginning to show more interest in what was going on, particularly when he had the chance to lead a group himself. His sculpts were usually comic, reflecting his attitude to the proceedings as a whole, but were often inventive. He would not commit himself when it came to feelings, however. It was hard to make him see that the purpose of miming the story of the creation of the world (Genesis I) was not an evangelical one: 'Now you're bringing religion in! That's not what we're *here* for' (Everything in its place).

Sessions 9–10. In the penultimate session, T at last found something that he could really see the point of, and contributed in an intelligent, and sympathetic way. In the 'animal psychodrama' various kinds of animals are used by group members to represent people in their own social and personal lives. Perhaps because of the simplicity and clarity that this game imposes upon our perception of other people, only allowing them to be 'like' one thing at a time, T found it interesting and stimulating. When we discussed its limitations afterwards he was still fascinated enough to take part seriously. In Session X he was asked to 'put himself in the shoes' of the husband of another group member. This was a role he could really understand and consequently identify with, and he responded well to the exercise.

In these last few sessions T showed that he was really quite willing to join in exercises he could understand the point of. This was the extent of his real participation, however, and he did not attempt to try anything new, except insofar as the experience of taking part at all in this kind of adventure in shared imagination was certainly new to him.

JP – Age 37

When she first came to the Day Hospital, J gave as her principal 'problem', 'trying to change the world and getting frustrated when I can't'. This, or the state of mind behind it, certainly seems to be a salient characteristic of her way of construing reality. J was born in Leicester. She never knew her natural father who died soon after her birth. Two years later her mother was married again, to a widower with one daughter, and it was this man whom J came to love and to depend on, rather than her mother. He has since died, but J's mother is still alive, living in the Midlands. Although she says she is not at all close to her mother, J certainly keeps in touch with her and sometimes goes to see her.

Because of her close relationship with her step-father, J's childhood was secure and happy. At the age of sixteen, however, her world was shattered when he left home for another woman. About the same time J became pregnant by her boy friend. Talking about these events, J gives a strong impression that she suffered more than her mother did as a result of the marital breakdown: 'I never really got on with her. She's not a very maternal person, and I'm the opposite. Mind you, she's married again now'. J married her boy friend and had two daughters by him. This 'shot-gun' marriage did not last, however, and the couple lived apart for some years before J met her present husband. She has now made friends with her first husband, after a period of hostility on his part. (J hates to be at odds with people and will always seek a reconciliation even if there has not been any real division, as there obviously was in this case. To be on good terms with her first husband means a great deal to her). Before she married her second husband, J moved in with him and changed her name to his by deed-poll before they moved first to the Midlands, where her next two children were born, and then to the North. At some stage in this itinerary, J began to develop the habit of drinking quite heavily. She says she can't remember exactly when this started, or what the immediate reasons for it may have been. Trying to keep so many potential enemies friendly, feeling responsible for breakdowns in communication, just trying to be everybody's mother – all these things must have exerted a strain. In addition, her present husband has been made redundant three times in the last few years, and her latest pregnancy, although emotionally welcome, was financially ill-advised. The heavy drinking certainly has something to do with what J describes as 'having to take the world on my back'. She says that she picks up ideas and feelings easily from other people, 'so that I find myself getting upset about all sorts of things'. What she sees on TV and reads in newspapers causes her a good deal of anguish: 'I just can't help applying it all to me. I get upset about things that aren't anything to do with me'. It seems that the drinking habit was a response to a general feeling of sadness on behalf of other people, an attempt to 'drown *their* sorrows', although, of course, they had now become J's sorrows. She says she did not intend to 'take up drinking as a way of coping with my problems'; it was to be 'only temporary, just to get me through a bad patch'. Intended to lift her out of the misery induced by other people's sufferings, the treatment only aggravated the malady.

This talent for empathy seems to fit in with J's overall personality. She is volatile, easily moved to tears and laughter, quick to pick up changes in emotional tone, quarrelsome and eager to please, and conscious of her appearance without really taking responsibility for it (perhaps she feels more responsible for others'). J is engulfed by the experiences of others so that whatever is happening to them seems to be happening to her too. She complains mildly about her husband, and also the married daughter who lives nearby, saying they are 'very soft-hearted, they cry easily'. They cannot supply those elements of firmness and strength that J senses she needs – although she does not say so. She subscribes to a long list of charities for relieving distressed people and animals. Her garden is full of the graves of dead pets.

J never really wanted to come to the drama therapy sessions. On each occasion, she would say 'do I really have to come?', and I would reply, 'no, but I'd like you to come', and she would come and join in, trying her best to take part as fully as she could. I assumed that this was a game, intended to reassure J that she was really wanted; however it turned out to be a genuine attempt to avoid having to attend the session: 'I really meant it.' J joined in because I said I would like her to. That is all I said, but with J it is enough. I particularly wanted her to come because of the part she played in the group, helping people to feel for others and understand what it was like to imagine you were somebody else.

But that's not difficult for you, is it?

– 'I'm there anyway'.

Did you really want to come?

– 'I was very apprehensive. I don't like people staring at me. It was extremely embarrassing, surrounded by people. I did not want to come. Some days were worse than others. I wanted an explanation of why we're doing it. What were you trying to achieve by doing it?' (I had explained to J that the exercises were put together to 'give people practice in relating to one another and using their imagination to see things from different points of view, so that they could understand themselves and other people better'. None of this seemed very relevant to J, who believed she could already see people's point of view painfully clearly).

You didn't like any of it?

– 'I didn't like getting involved in things and then having to stop. The parts I enjoyed were when it got interesting. I appreciated the trust exercises, because physical contact is hard for me, and I got better as I went along. I got to trust people more. When I looked back on the weeks I found that I had a small amount of confidence. I still don't understand the whole meaning of the exercise, but things did fit into place towards the end of the drama therapy'.

J sums up her feelings: 'At first I did not enjoy drama therapy at all. I felt silly, this is not what I need. I do not want to be with others. My problems were mine, I do not like to touch anyone else. I liked Roger and Mary (the therapists) but I objected to being a sheep. Later I began to realise what it all meant, but I still think we should talk more. I do not like role play. It helps to think that all of us in the group do benefit by being together... I feel very pleased when the session is over and I understand what it is all about'. Urged to be more explicit about her reasons for not liking role play, J said 'I don't want my thoughts inside someone else's head and someone else's thoughts inside my head'. This seems to suggest that she finds it difficult to discriminate between different modes of mental experience, and does not like being 'put to the test'. Her role playing was effective and convincing, but painful to her. Would it have become less painful with practice?

Sessions 1–3. J showed little difficulty in making sense of the exercises. Only one member of the group scored higher in 'sorting according to personal characteristics', and J talked freely and openly in front of the others. (She admits she has little difficulty in talking to individuals, but this was to a group.)

Session 4. J left early. She gave no explanation at the time. Afterwards she said she 'hadn't felt up to it'. She did not attend the next session.

Sessions 5 and 7. J took part in all the exercises, usually asking what was the point of things, but appearing to enjoy anything which involved using her imagination.

Session 8. J began the session in her usual way, saying 'do I have to come?', but began smiling during the first exercise, and seemed to enjoy doing the sculpting. Her sculpts were very expressive, both when she herself was the subject, and when she was moulding someone else. She was able to talk effectively about this.

Session 9. The 'animal psychodrama' seems to have seized J's imagination, providing an opportunity for involvement of a 'safe' kind. Her ability to see herself as someone else and 'take on' other people's feelings could be publicly demonstrated, while the nature of the exercise as a game, a wholly contingent reality, provided a clear indication of the division between her real and assumed identities. She could invade someone else without being engulfed by them.

Session 10. Talking about last week's session J said 'I still feel it's nerve-racking, but I can understand the point of it when I look back on it. It was silly, you did it for a laugh, then you got involved'. I asked J if she would like to use real people for the psychodrama, instead of toy animals? She said she wouldn't mind having a go at this, so we pretended that somebody was sitting in an empty chair. Would we like to say something to this person? Would we like to put ourselves in their place and talk back to us? Several people did this but no one as convincingly as J (who spoke to, and then as, an imaginary critic of drama therapy!).

Moving on to the family sculpt, we concentrated on the families of two people present, one of which was the therapist's (in order to give people an idea of the kinds of thing involved in this kind of sculpt). J took part in both sculpts playing the part of members of the families. Afterwards she told the therapist 'I didn't do my family because it was so like yours. I felt involved'. Evidently the identity of this exercise as simply an exercise was not sufficiently clear to J; she could not distance herself from what was going on. On the other hand, she has certainly gained in self-confidence since the first sessions, although she is still more assertive 'in role' than out of it.

EG – Age 26

Although an attractive young woman with an interesting approach to life – she usually manages to supply an element of novelty to any conversation or group discussion she is involved in – E considers herself to be an almost total outcast: 'I'm rubbish'. Her viewpoint is extremely individualistic, and her attitude aggressive. She emphatically does not care if people find her 'odd'. At the same time, she clings to her independence of outlook. An only child, E is firmly established as an observer rather than a participant, critical of everything that goes on around her, more critical of herself than anyone else, with the exception of her mother.

E's mother is a teacher in a secondary school, an intelligent and capable woman who runs the household more or less single-handed. ('My husband decided a long time ago that I should make the decisions'.) It was E's mother who decided that E should seek psychiatric help, despite E's objection to having to associate with 'mad' people, an objection which she frequently repeated during the course of the drama therapy sessions, carefully excepting those present from any such criticism. The doctor who first inter-viewed her on her arrival at the Day Hospital records that her attitude was 'self-deni-grating, wholly negative. She is unco-operative at home, and has a bad relationship with her mother. She stays in bed when not working'; and indeed E's job as a temporary secretary seems to fit in very well with her determination to 'do her own thing'. If she doesn't feel like working she simply doesn't bother to look for a job.

Unfortunately this arrangement is not as satisfactory as in theory it should have been, even from E's point of view. E complains of her isolation. Whether or not this was originally self-imposed it now causes her a great deal of distress. She wants to share her thoughts and feelings with others, but finds she has not got the language of common ideas and experiences to do this. Her language is not sufficiently flexible and well articulated, flexible enough to subsume other ways of looking at life, articulate enough to present her own construct system in ways which make it accessible to others. When she says, as she frequently does, 'I just can't talk to people' she means that she can't listen to them properly either. The ground of relationship, what we have called the interchange of engulfment and individuation, has not properly developed or has been drastically affected. 'I'm a mess, nothing is straightforward,' E says.

This awareness of being separated from the source of life comes across quite strongly: 'I don't seem able to make relationships. It's as if I've never grown up. I'm not real.'

Questioned about the relationships she had made during her life she said they were 'few and far between, usually very shallow.' The idea of other people is a threat, although 'when it comes to it, I can usually manage to get on with them. It's the *idea*, you see'. As the admitting doctor noticed during the first interview, E frequently talks about death. This is usually death as a condition rather than as an event: 'She is fascinated by death and suicide as ideas'. In my own conversations with E, I have received the impression that she thinks the condition of being dead might give her a sort of reality which eludes her while she is alive. She is fascinated by the state of mind that people would be in, faced by the death of this person about whom they understood so little, and *whom they could never get through to while she was alive*. Death is a statement that even they could understand. What, E wonders, would their response be? 'What will they say when I've gone?' Something relevant at last, perhaps! The concentration upon death seems to be a reflection of E's 'negativity' rather than a real desire to kill herself. For her the world is an empty place, devoid of the meaning necessary to make any course of action, even suicide, really significant. She complains of 'thinking too much', yet her thoughts are unorganised, and this is what frightens her most, as she feels herself in danger of being overwhelmed by a shapeless mass of ideas and feelings she cannot control, a threateningly formless universe which dominates her while eluding her efforts to come to terms with it and make a kind of sense out of chaos. Because E is able to envisage a state of affairs in which this conflict is resolved and she is at peace with herself and other people, she says she feels she is caught between two extremes, a lovingly simple view of life and a present reality which is not simple at all, but terrifyingly formless.

For E all relationships tend to reproduce the one she has with her parents, one of mutual misunderstanding and absence of acceptance. The people she went to school with were 'all two-faced, and nobody liked me. Nobody ever likes me.' E would very much like to be liked, in a straightforward uncomplicated way, without having to compromise and make allowances and 'see things from somebody else's point of view'. She dare not look too closely into other people in case she finds out what they really think about her – they couldn't possibly *like* her. So she withdraws and 'keeps her powder dry'.

E is very much aware that she is doing this, and it makes her feel cowardly and impotent. 'If I got stuck in, I know I could change my life.' At the moment, however, she is continuing to keep people at a distance, apart from one or two friends who are able to make her feel she is 'not so horrible'. Her extreme dislike of the Thought Disorder Test may possibly be due to a fear of drawing conclusions about other people because it might lead to a reciprocal invasion of privacy, rather than a straightforward inability to categorise systematically. Perhaps the two things are connected! She says that she feels 'calm and relaxed' in other people's company, but that she finds social occasions 'unsettling'. 'Relaxed' and 'on edge' at the same time, she appears to be talking nonsense about herself until one realises that what she is describing is a situation of almost complete detachment. E imputes to other people certain ideas and attitudes towards herself and these cause her concern and give rise to resentment. At the same time, however, she feels herself to be impregnable within her own chosen persona, and is able to present herself, to herself as well as other people, as poised and relaxed. She doesn't find this kind of 'showing off' very satisfactory and longs for more genuine encounters, which is why she goes on seeking out ways of meeting people even though it makes her feel 'on edge'...

E treated the idea of joining the drama therapy sessions with a good deal of disdain. She had already refused to carry out the Thought Disorder Test, although, once pressure was removed, she decided to go along with the rest and do it herself. This set the pattern for most of the ten weeks of the programme itself: E would hang back and then join in, attracted and repelled by the group's liveliness. Eventually, in the penultimate session, she found a place for her own feelings, an opportunity to express herself to people who had proved themselves willing to listen.

> *What, in general, did you think of the drama therapy, E?*
>
> – 'I thought it was all stupid. Pointless. A waste of time'.
>
> *You seemed to be enjoying some of it, though.*
>
> – 'Well, you join in, don't you? Some of it was all right, I suppose'.
>
> *Was there anything that you did really think was all right?*
>
> – 'I liked the family thing. That was good'. (She grins at the memory.)

Sessions 1–5. E joined in the exercises, but without enthusiasm. Her finger painting was harsh in content and execution, (she refused to say what it represented for her), as were her string pictures (Sessions II and III), and her miming (Session IV). Having expressed the violence of her feelings in these indirect ways, she remained silent and refused to comment: 'What I have done, I have done'.

Session 6. E was very much aware of the reality of opposing emotions demonstrated in the individual and group sculpts, and was able to put something of this into words in the exercise which followed. '*People* make me angry'. 'I hate *myself*; 'coming to this place makes me *ashamed*. People talk about you when they know you come here'. (This last remark led to a heated discussion, with a good deal of anger from other members of the group, as well as E.)

Sessions 7 and 8. E found difficulty in thinking of three things about herself that she liked, and finally only produced one, 'my typing'. Among many alternatives, she selected 'my appearance', 'my uselessness', and 'me', as things she would like to get rid of. She was obviously bored by the sculpts, which provided no kind of challenge, except that of inventing variations upon her one all-consuming emotion, anger. The idea of finding alternatives to this from within her own experience utterly confounded her. (Session VIII).

Sessions 9 and 10. By now E was expressing, and sharing, her anger much more effectively than at the beginning of the programme, when her feelings were closely confined or turned in on herself. There were no longer times in which she wept silently to herself, as she had in the first few sessions. Her active participation and involvement in the groups reached a climax in the 'family sculpt' in Session X. Fortunately other members of the group were able to identify with a good deal of the material provided by E, so that she was able to bring her family to life in psychodramatic form in a way which plainly had great personal meaning for her. Group members recognised so much of their own experience in the scenario provided by E that they were able to respond to their cues in ways which provided her with a living picture of how things were, and also – because each person's viewpoint, while remaining sympathetic to E's, was slightly different from hers – with a whole range of alternative attitudes to, and interpretations of, the interpersonal situation in which she perceived herself to be enmeshed. When E battered away at her 'mother', her anger no longer deprived her of words, and those she could not find were discovered for her by others. Other people supported her, too, when the time came for her to put herself in her mother's place and let something of her long-suppressed love for her mother find expression at last. The dramatic structure and the flexibility of the role-reversal and role-exchanging techniques allowed the other members of the group to help E explore parts of herself she had not dared to approach for a long time, parts which had to do with identifying with the experiences of other people as living, breathing, vulnerable individuals rather than as symbols of undifferentiated hate, love, fear, guilt etc., pre-emptive constructs which forced every element of personal awareness to conform to their outline.

DT – Age 63

D lives with her aged mother in a council flat. Her father died 16 years ago, at the age of 82. He had previously had a heart attack, and had required nursing for several years before he died. Before they moved to this town D and her mother had lived in the same house for forty years. D still misses 'our little house', and finds the flat claustrophobic. The house had had no bathroom and was unsuitable for looking after elderly people in, but the neighbours were helpful and supportive, even to the extent of sharing their bathroom and toilet facilities. Unfortunately since moving to their flat D and her mother have lost touch with these people, and with almost everyone else they had known. In fact, they have no visitors to their new home at all. D misses her two uncles especially, both of whom are now dead. A cousin of whom she was particularly fond has emigrated with her family to Australia.

As a young woman D worked at a local factory, making children's toys and games, a job she enjoyed very much. She is left-handed, due to a weakness in her right arm. Although she manages very well, to the extent of being able to carry out delicate embroidery, she blames her mother for the fact that her right hand is weaker than her left one: 'if my mother hadn't been too shy as a young woman to take me to the doctor's, I wouldn't be like this'.

D's world is very much taken up with her relationship with her mother. This has not always been as painful as it has become during the last few years. D says that the two of them lived happily together in the days when they shared the family home. 'In those days', D says, 'we were very close'. Nowadays things are different. Moving into a flat has emphasised D's role as companion/housekeeper. Tasks that were once shared are now left completely to her. What was once a shared responsibility is now a personal burden, and during the past year D has become increasingly alienated from the flat and everything associated with it. Her mother's growing forgetfulness has started to irritate her, as does the old lady's tendency to complain about her various aches and pains – 'she used to be so straight and proud, and now she's started to stoop'. These signs of increasing age in her mother are a source of considerable distress to D. After all, her mother is the only other person to whom she is able to relate on a genuinely personal level.

In the last few weeks things have started to get considerably worse. D finds she can no longer hold a conversation with her mother: 'she says I always talk a load of rubbish'. D's way of coping with this is to stand and scream. It was this that led to her being admitted to hospital. After some weeks as an in-patient, during which her anxiety about her mother increased, D was allowed home on condition that she attends the Day Hospital. She says that she enjoys coming here, and she certainly joins in the activities provided. She is friendly towards the other patients, bringing newcomers into the social group and taking the initiative in sharing experiences with others. On one occasion she demonstrated several new card games to the group. The Day Hospital seems to be an acceptable compromise between having to spend all day with her mother and cutting loose from her altogether. When she was an in-patient she was extremely anxious about how her mother was managing in the flat, and a visit home confirmed her suspicions that her mother was not able to cope without her. Coming to the Day Hospital, however, provides an outlet for her sociable personality. D is much more gregarious than her quiet, rather old-maidish appearance suggests.

How did you feel about the drama therapy?

– 'I didn't want to do it at first. I felt poorly that day, but I didn't want to be left out, so I joined in. It wasn't bad, really. A bit strange'.

You found it strange. Anything else?

– 'I enjoyed it when I got used to it. Some of the games were fun'.

So what was the point of it, do you think?

– 'I think it was to get you used to working things out together. To get you used to seeing things from other people's point of view'.

Did it help you in any way, do you think?

– 'I got a few things off my chest'.

Session 1. During this session D spent most of the time sitting down at the side of the room, although she did get up for a mirroring exercise. She said that she had an upset stomach, and that this was why she couldn't join in more actively. I got the impression that she quite enjoyed the session.

Sessions 2 and 3. D is a rather fastidious lady, and I expected her to refuse to use finger paints. I certainly didn't think she would produce so imaginative and free a painting as she did – delicate, colourful and artistic. She filled the whole sheet with light finger strokes; 'This is how I feel, hopeful but confused'. She did not enjoy the 'blind walk', finding it difficult to put herself in someone else's hands to such an extent, although she was more at ease when she was doing the leading. (She said she thought she had been 'hypnotised' when she was being led, and she didn't like this.)

Sessions 4 and 5. D joined in all the exercises, obediently rather than enthusiastically. She was still finding it all rather confusing, but she didn't want to be left out, and enjoyed being involved with the other group members. The more active exercises made her feel nervous, perhaps because of the presence of younger people who were more agile than she.

Session 6. This was a good session for everyone involved. As the other group members began to enjoy themselves, D relaxed very noticeably, and started to use her body in a much more expressive way. She was particularly forthcoming in the final 'feelings' exercise, describing the kind of situation that made her feel angry: 'when people won't try and understand what you mean, and make out you mean something you don't'.

Sessions 7, 8. D joined in more enthusiastically now. She was able to express emotion more easily and to cope with other people's feelings without embarrassment. She described how her love for her father had grown during his final illness. She enjoyed

Session VIII particularly, and seemed to have an air of serenity and poise during the sculpting which contrasted strongly with her initial uncertainty.

Sessions 9 and 10. This feeling of serenity continued through both the final sessions. D joined in the 'family sculpt' (the most testing of the exercises), speaking sensitively 'in character' as someone she had never met and with whom she had little in common except in the shared life of the imagination. It was surprising to see how someone who had lived so sheltered a life for so long was able to 'come out of herself' to such an extent. She is still very shy, of course, and needs a lot of reassurance about her ability to do things.

These people were all members of an introductory course in drama therapy (the one described in the previous chapter). In order to achieve some idea of whether or not the therapy had affected their ways of seeing the world they were tested on Construct Theory lines before and after the course. The actual measure was that provided by the Grid Test for Thought Disorder (Bannister and Fransella, 1966). This was chosen because of its flexibility – it is able to distinguish tendencies towards depressed ways of thinking as well as confused or 'over-loose' construing. Another reason for its suitability is that it concerns the way we see people; its actual subject matter consists of photographs of individual men and women which have to be related to one another. The test measures the INTENSITY of the degree to which ideas (constructs) are correlated, and CONSISTENCY of performance in doing this.[1] However the information provided by the test goes beyond the computation of scores for intensity and consistency. By looking at individual 'grids' and noting particular correlations of constructs it is possible to build up a picture of the way someone's mind functions – not only their overall ability to 'make' sense but the individual kinds of sense they make, their personal system of associations. 'Reading' the grids in such a way produced the following results:

TM This person was a tight construer, lacking in flexibility of thought. The nature of the constructs supplied in the test does not show how limited T's repertoire may really be, but the results indicated a lack of association between clusters of constructs, suggesting an equally inefficient way of anticipating events as that of an over-loose construer. Certainly, from the things he said during the interviews and his behaviour and attitude in the group, T showed signs of having the simple, relatively inflexible construct system associated with a clinical diagnosis of obsessional neurosis 'characterised by the compulsion to dwell on certain themes' (Bannister & Fransella, 1986: 150, I). The tightening is *exclusive.* Bannister and Fransella suggest that 'the obsessional had so constricted their construing of the environment that the only part of their system with tight structure was that to do with their obsessional thoughts and acts.' The results indicated that this occurred here, suggesting a way of construing reality which is inflexible and limited in scope, what Kelly calls an 'impermeable' system, making it hard for an individual to change his or her views in the light of new, contradictory, evidence. T's post-treatment results suggested a better articulated system than his pre-treatment one. Drama therapy seems to have helped him 'elaborate and build up constructs outside his symptom-based system' (Bannister & Fransella 1986: 152). Tom left hospital as soon as he could, which was immediately after the programme finished. He had had enough, he said.

JP According to the criteria established by Bannister and Fransella, J's thinking was disordered when the programme began. At the end of the ten sessions she was found to be thinking more clearly and consistently although her constructs tended still to be negative, reflecting her preoccupation with suffering and her lack of confidence in herself. J always seemed to have difficulty with boundaries: reality and fantasy overlapped considerably, as did people, places and times. She was conscious of a tendency to 'live other people's lives for them' (J's phrase) and seemed almost swamped by the accumulation of feelings this created. J always resisted attending sessions, even the last ones, which she said she enjoyed. It was the urge to please someone else, in this case the therapist, that drew her into the group. The last session found her tougher and more determined than before, having found the determination to cut down on her drinking. J attended a continuation drama therapy group until discharged from hospital some months later.

EG The sessions had a tightening effect on a very loose construct system, so that by the end E had, technically, ceased to be thought disordered. There was always a tendency towards hostility revealing a determination to cling on to the vague outline of an independent selfhood that distinguished her from her mother. On the other hand, much of the anger was directed inwards; it was as if E had internalised her mother's contempt of herself. Throughout the sessions E gave the impression that she was the victim of a global campaign against herself. The results of the Thought Disorder Test showed that she saw herself as cheated by a mean world. Everything was very threatening but extremely vague – there was no tight system as there would have been with paranoia. Drama therapy went at least some way towards personalising E's imagination, helping her to sort out what she really did feel, about whom she felt it, and why. There was something pathetic about E's unfocused rage which engaged the sympathies of the group. E said it was 'wonderful to be treated like a person'. She left hospital soon afterwards without joining another group.

DT D was almost completely preoccupied with her elderly mother. An increase in the degree of organisation in her construct system after the ten drama therapy sessions represented an even more committed awareness than before, but one possessing greater openness and resilience. The actual sessions revealed, however, a definite process of the widening and deepening of D's relationship to the group. As the dramatic process became more familiar as a safe means of self-disclosure, D allowed more of her deeply held feelings and attitudes to surface. Perhaps someone of her generation was bound to be doubtful of the wisdom of letting other people in on private matters, particularly a group. Round about the third session D opened out like a butterfly from its chrysalis. Perhaps her experience had made her take a new look at her relationship with her mother; the post session test results showed a strong new correlation between ideas of unselfishness and stupidity! Had she been too unselfish? Was it, in the long run, the best way of caring? While she remained, she stayed a member of a group.

These are four histories taken more or less at random from the records usually kept of drama therapy group members. More comprehensive information is usually available about the sessions themselves, and various systems exist for codifying relationships and states of mind within the group process itself. There is no real substitute for a person's own picture of him or herself, just as there is no denying the importance of the process recording as a way of conveying the quality of an interpersonal event (see Appendix 1). Initial interviews take place before a programme of sessions begins, and descriptive accounts of the actual process, either in words or symbols, necessarily follow sessions, and after programmes have been completed. Certainly there are no interruptions for note-taking of any kind during the sessions themselves.

Notes

1. The procedure for administering this is given in Appendix 2, along with a diagrammatic summary of the results of the investigation.

Chapter 7

'Capturing the Image'

Different kinds of healing require different criteria for assessing improvement, different methods of validation. For behavioural analysts, the success of a cure will depend on the degree of change within particular behaviour patterns, the generalisation of specific responses, the extinction of maladaptive conditioned operants and so forth, all things that are readily identified and conveniently measured (indeed, they have been devised precisely in order to be so). Other schools of psychotherapy validate their approach in terms of the degree to which a patient's or client's way of looking at himself and the world has changed for the better. Effective psychotherapy is considered to be that which provides an appropriate setting for the kinds of personal relationship between therapist and client which the latter can acknowledge as a source of strength, confidence and psychological repose for the other relationships in his or her life (Bannister, 1980). This does not mean, of course, that the *effects* of drama therapy cannot be assessed in any kind of systematic way. Drama therapy alters the ways in which people look at the world, themselves and other people, and its results may be studied by examining changes in behaviour and perception which take place as a result of things which happen to the individual within the dramatherapeutic situation. The 'unscientific' aspect is the inability of the method to be specific about the precise conditions under which such changes occur so that these conditions may be exactly reproduced, and change reliably predicted.

The psychodramatic tradition lays a great deal of stress on the personal testimony of the client. 'In psychodrama especially', says Moreno, 'the full involvement of the actor in the act is a regular procedure, and emphasis is continually placed upon a subjectivistic frame of reference to the extreme...' (1972: 215).[1] This kind of 'existential validation' is obviously more vague than the 'objective' criteria required by mechanistic psychology. It should not be assumed that it is less truthful about the human condition, however. The concept of human experience as a kind of universal drama is fundamental to psychodrama and informs the various kinds of drama therapy which are derived from it. Drama therapy and psychodrama do not make *use* of drama, in the way that certain kinds of psychother-apy make use of simulation, role-play and modelling; they *are* drama. That is to say, they present the entire psychotherapeutic enterprise as a conscious drama, a piece of theatre in which everybody, whether they be clients or therapists, is playing his or her particular role. An important characteristic of drama therapy is that everyone present takes part; people cannot help participating, because the role of non-participant is even more noticeable (and constitutes an act in itself) than that of the person who joins in willingly with the others.

From one point of view this makes the sort of judgements arrived at in this kind of 'therapy of total participation' actually more scientific than clinical investigations which aim at 'scientific detachment'. It has been pointed out by philosophers of science that the kind of scientific objectivity aimed at by many psychologists is in fact a myth, and an outworn one, too. The 'desperate craving to represent scientific knowledge as impersonal', says Michael Polanyi 'has come to threaten the position of science itself. This self-contradiction stems from a misguided intellectual passion – a passion for achieving absolutely impersonal knowledge which, being unable to recognise any persons, presents us with a picture of the universe in which we ourselves are absent' (1958: 60). In other words, it is a universe which is totally unscientific, because there is nobody in it to take a scientific attitude about it, as everybody has withdrawn from the field of study, in order to observe it with perfect objectivity. As Kant pointed out, there is no way in which we *can* draw conclusions about things apart from the way that we *do* draw them; in other words as a living part of the very conclusions we are drawing, we are deeply, inextricably and fundamentally involved in, and affected by, the data we are studying. When this data is the life and experience of men and women like ourselves, as it is in psychology and psychotherapy, our intellectual impartiality is bound to be more than ordinarily suspect.

In any case, science depends more on the communication of experience than it does upon any kind of 'scientific impartiality'. As Smail says, 'the conviction which scientific statements carry…stems not from checking them from an outside, 'objective' reality (which is an illusion), but from internal experience… Scientific truth becomes possible as a concept because we happen to share certain important areas of our experience' (1978: 69, 71). When the scientific enterprise in which we are involved concerns the business of promoting psychological well-being, the function of *sharing*, whether we call it 'insight', 'involvement', 'empathy', 'the cycle of individuation and engulfment' or 'tele' (Moreno's term), becomes more salient than ever.

Drama therapy is itself an open-ended, divergent experience, one best evaluated in terms of the uniqueness of what has been produced rather than by the application of a common standard of direction and degree of behavioural change. As Eisner says, however, 'scientific procedures are not the only forms through which human understanding is secured and scientific methods are not the only ways through which human influence can be confidently created' (1985: 103). Any attempt to think critically about drama therapy should take account of the context in which this kind of activity takes place. One of the most important things about this kind of activity is the relationship between activity and setting, foreground and background, which makes the overall effect highly context-specific. The freedom and spontaneity of the sessions contrasts with the highly technical background of the modern hospital or clinic, and particularly with the strict regulation of responses required for good performance in clinical tests, drawing its particular significance from the contrast. In this sense standardised testing plays an important purpose as part of the background against which the drama therapy exercises stand out as expressions of freedom and inventiveness. Some of the people who took part in the programme described in the text certainly saw it in this way. Whilst enjoying the actual sessions, they resisted the change of role from group member to experimental subject.

The principal objection to the use of standardised tests to evaluate open ended or expressive activity lies in the inability of nomothetic techniques for the measurement of behaviour change to take proper account of the most important kind of datum produced by such activity – in other words, the uniqueness of the individual response. Scientific assessment depends on the manipulation of groups of people whose combined scores represent no identifiable single reality. Artistic creativity, on the other hand, generates symbolic forms which themselves present in a direct and *immediate* way an idea, image or feeling which resides within rather than outside the symbol, and is consequently *itself* rather than the reduction of itself by being translated into something else. The problem is always to find evaluation procedures which correspond to the process under inspection without reducing the process to a form in which it would fit the available research procedures.

This was, and remains, exceedingly difficult. The main reason has already been suggested. It subsists in the nature of drama therapy as art rather than science: drama therapy uses metaphor to express the intangible quality of human experience, and metaphor cannot be adequately described in any other terms than itself. Indeed it has been observed that interpretations of what is actually happening in therapy are more like aesthetic than scientific judgements precisely because they aim at structuring experiential data in order to give it meaning within its own terms rather than trying to explain it in terms of something outside itself (Cheshire, 1975: 3, 86). This is *acted* metaphor; in other words you really need to see it, or even to participate in it yourself. Otherwise you are left with measuring an artificially contrived 'final effect' without really studying the process by which such an effect may have been brought about. The descriptions represent a kind of metaphor of the writer's experience of the interaction in which he found himself involved.

When scientific measurement is inappropriate, artistic criticism may prove helpful. In art 'precision is not necessarily a function of quantification' (Eisner, 1985: 101).[2] Following Eisner, there is room for a concept of 'therapeutic criticism' – how to judge whether a treatment modality has had an effect *in terms of the modality* rather than according to criteria imported from elsewhere which are likely to affect what we see by inappropriately angling how we see it ('The tests we use are not simply neutral entities, but have distinctive effects on the quality of our perception and upon our understanding' – Eisner, 1985: 114). In evaluating a drama therapy session some such considerations as the following might be appropriate:

- to what extent did the group create its own world?
- how conscious were those involved of moving across an invisible line separating the drama therapy session from the ordinary world?
- how difficult was it for individuals to 'de-brief' and leave this specific world behind them?
- how successful was the drama in establishing its own laws about personal identity? Were people free to 'become' one another in it?
- did people feel free to experiment with changing reality *dramatically*?
- what about relationships among the group members themselves? Were people 'left outside'? If they were, was this by their own choice or because the rest of the group decided it should be so?
- were there any examples of 'narrator effect', in which one or more people straddled the dividing line between two worlds, commenting on one in terms of the other? If there were, how successful were they in doing it, and what was its effect on the session?
- how did things 'go' for individuals? For the group as a whole? Did anything memorable happen for anyone? Do individuals feel happier or sadder, freer or more restrained?
- what comments were made afterwards? Immediately? Some days later?

These are the kinds of insight one would expect to gain from an adequate account of drama therapy. Such an account would have to be imaginative, and even to some extent poetic. It would have to use language in a flexible way so that it was sometimes figurative and sometimes prosaic. The aim would be to get as near the experience of movement and speech as possible. What we are attempting here is to use a means of expression which is sympathetic to or compatible with its subject matter.

In the following accounts of drama therapy I have attempted this kind of 'therapeutic criticism'. My aim has been to put down on paper what is actually going on in a particular session. Obviously this has been done at what is in some ways a very superficial level.

From a whole range of standpoints – sociological, psychological, biological, aesthetic – all sorts of other things were happening during the sessions. Looked at like this, what follows are woefully inadequate account of the occasions, because they are only the impression of a single person, and not at all objective, as he was himself a member of the group.

An impression is precisely what we need, however. The aim is to get a feeling of what the occasion was like, because this is really the only way one can judge whether or not it has *'worked'*, and whether it will be internalised as an experience and used for future living. What is presented here is a complete event, 'a cultural network saturated with meaning'. To isolate particular aspects of it, drawing out the threads that constitute the whole, is to distort the pattern. It is only possible to tell what it is really like, what is really happening, by being there yourself – and by being involved. If you can't be there you may perhaps be enabled to experience something of the nature and quality of the event so far as this can be transmitted by a sympathetic and imaginative description of it.

First session

The setting is a hall in the Day Hospital, roughly a hundred feet by thirty or forty. Architecturally, it is 1960s functional, with a most unfunctional stage at one end, not practical for drama of any kind, certainly not drama therapy. The hall is airy and clean. It has recently been re-decorated. This afternoon it seems a bit dull, because the curtains have been drawn over the windows, shutting out the afternoon sunshine.

The group consists of ten people to begin with – eight women and two men. Three of these, two women and a man, are leaders. Another member, a woman, joins the group about five minutes after the start of proceedings. It is hard for the leaders to get things going, as people seem jumpy and nervous. They are not exactly unco-operative, but are finding it hard to concentrate on anything for more than a moment at a time. Roger, one of the leaders, suggests that we pull the curtains back. The general feeling however is that it would be better to turn the lights on. Another leader, Mary, says she's feeling particularly anti-drama therapy this afternoon. Conversation while we're waiting to begin is jerky, moving by fits and starts. This may be because people are feeling apprehensive about next week's session, a week today, when a T/V company are visiting the Day Hospital and intend to film some of the session. Surprisingly, no-one mentions this. The sheer size of the hall magnifies nervousness.

We begin the session by dividing into two groups and lining up on opposite sides of the hall. Let's conquer the space – and the anxiety that fills it – by trying to outshout each other. One group yells 'yes' and the other group screams 'no'. People enjoy doing this and we make a lot of noise. So long as we remain as groups nobody holds back. When we move to the middle line of the hall, however, and start yelling at the person opposite us, Janet gets worried and refuses to do it any more. The group loses its cohesion, as people exchange roles, shouting 'yes' and 'no' backwards and forwards indiscriminately. Roger, one of the leaders, tries to gain control. Unfortunately he isn't sure of the plan he and the others have worked out beforehand for the running of the group. By this time people are enjoying themselves too much to pay much attention to his rather vague suggestion that it might be time to 'move on to something else'. Mary, another of the leaders, shepherds everyone into a circle and explains the next exercise. People are to think of a feeling or an attitude of mind and stand as if they were statues representing or embodying it. She uses the word 'embody' and shows what she means by twisting herself round to express 'hidden-ness'. Mary's instructions are clear and her example is a vivid one. She begins to exert her particular influence on the group, one of firmness, and clarity. Roger follows her example, miming 'inspiration'. This draws forth a rather derisory comment, and people laugh. Obviously we would rather fool than work this afternoon. The exercise gets off to a slow start. After a few minutes it gathers pace, as people find a way of harnessing their nervous energy. After threatening to get out of hand, it slows down and becomes thoughtful. The feelings expressed are all negative, though the ways in which they are expressed are inventive, and there is a good deal of laughter. Towards the end of this section people begin spontaneously to help one another with their mimes.

When everybody has tried this, Roger suggests that they should go round the circle again. He explains that everybody has chosen rather gloomy feelings to portray, and 'we need some cheerful, positive ones for what we're going to do next...'. At this point he is prevented from saying what this is going to be by Mary, who mutters something about 'giving the game away'. People are, understandably, less spontaneous in their creations this time, but everyone seems to be concentrating hard. Lynda shares her feelings about the prospect of a new grandchild, choosing 'a sense of beauty' as the feeling she wants to portray. For the first time during the session itself anxiety about next week's T/V ordeal comes to the surface: Pat says she can't think of a positive feeling, she feels too nervous about next week. Someone says 'we're all in it together, Pat', and Pat grins and mimes 'friendly'. The group goes on to construct individual 'sculpts' in which each member uses the various feelings portrayed by members of the group in order to build up a composite picture of him or herself, 'myself as I am', or 'myself as I'd like to be'. We widen the circle to give more space in the middle, and people set about doing this game systematically, some choosing to do the first, some the second. The atmosphere is rather flat, as if people are just going through the motions, not really enjoying it or feeling much at all. Janet refuses an invitation from Roger to join in. She says 'I want to be the opposite of myself, but I'm not going to do it'. Roger says 'I know you'd like confidence. We all think that's the only thing you lack, Janet, don't we?' Most people say they agree with it. Spurred on by this – as it seems to her – outrageous remark, Janet sets up her personal sculpt, putting in 'adamant', 'in control', and 'angry'. This is definitely, she says, 'how I'd like to be'. Jean, a very restrained and rather reserved middle aged woman, chooses 'drunk', and 'degenerate', because 'that's the complete opposite of me, and it'd be a change'.

Sensing a growing feeling of interest and excitement in the group, Mary suggests that we build up a picture of the entire group, using all the feelings and ideas that have evolved and putting all the poses together. What does the group mean to us? If we want a feeling we haven't mentioned we can get someone to do a sculpt of it for us, and we can include this. Slowly and tentatively we start to do this. It seems a very serious thing to be doing, more significant in some ways than individual sculpts. After all you can always say, like Janet, 'I can't think of anything'. People seem to feel a powerful urge to join in. Two of the kitchen staff pass through the hall on the way to the room where they change out of their orange overalls. They seem yards rather than feet away. Attention is focused on this part of the room, which seems lighter than the rest, but this must be a subjective impression, a kind of optical illusion. Again, humour comes in to lower the emotional temperature: Janet, seeing Roger take up a striking pose as 'inspired', calls out 'Oh look, isn't he lovely'; (This is funny because it's so uncharacteristic of Janet!) The final sculpt, presenting the group as it feels itself to be contains the following elements: 'In control', 'friendly', 'embarrassed', 'close', 'modest', 'energetic', 'humorous', 'reluctant', 'trustful', 'inspired', 'generous', 'out-going', 'understanding'. When we're all gathered together in the centre in our various interweaved poses Myra says 'we've forgotten "sharing"'. People say 'Oh yes', or 'Yes, we have'. Myra says, 'It's funny, you never get a feeling like this anywhere else'. Madge says 'You wouldn't do it anywhere else, I suppose'. We break our poses, putting our arms round one another's shoulders, and move in for a 'group hug' before saying goodbye. Slowly we begin to sway, first left, then right, then left again, then right again… Nobody knows who started the movement, just as we don't know who began the humming which rises and falls, filling the whole hall with sound. Everybody is smiling. Drama therapy is over for this week.

This has been a mixed-up session, alternating between fast and slow, boring and exciting. Sparked by Mary's idea, the last part certainly 'took off', and drama therapy suddenly began to seem a joyful celebratory thing. Individuals used the group sculpt as a way of speaking up for themselves and one another. It became a kind of moving sculpture as we moved in and out enjoying our presence within the whole. The ideas which the leaders had brought to the session seemed at one point to limit the group's spontaneity. In fact they provided a safe, rather dull background for individuality to emerge against. The group took over the structure provided by the leaders and evolved a new one which it could use as a jumping-off point rather than a place to hide.

In the light of our criteria for criticising drama therapy, we can say that this group 'created its own world'. It established its own pragmatic rules about personal identity. *Ad hoc* as these were, they carried powerful implications about the *ad hoc* nature of social roles. Personality was seen, and for a short time lived, as changeable and interchangeable. On this occasion nobody was left outside the group, or acted as narrator to what was going on. At least two people made discoveries about themselves which they mentioned later on, when the session was over. In general, people felt happier and behaved more freely.

Second session

The setting is the same as before. This time the group is completely new to drama therapy. It consists of four young women aged between twenty-five and thirty, (Vicky, Joan, Una and Dawn), an older woman in her mid-sixties (Elsie) and three middle aged men (Tom, George, Cyril). To begin with they stand in a cluster at one side of the hall, too nervous to leave one another, not even daring to sit down on the many chairs ranged along the wall. When the therapist comes in they begin to drift away, as though caught doing something that is not allowed. The therapist suggests they 'might like to get some chairs so we can sit in a circle'. They do this, arranging the chairs so that the men sit on one side and the women the other. The therapist says she thinks it might be a good idea if people were to get up and move around a bit 'so you're sitting in a different chair'. One of the men, Tom, says 'can't we stay where we are, Rose?' Rose smiles at him, and after a moment's pause, he moves to another chair. When everyone is more or less settled, Rose starts to say something about what is going to happen. 'This is the first of ten sessions we're going to be having. We're going to find ways of getting to know each other better. We shall be using our imagination to help us to do this. Nobody has to take part if they don't want to. If you leave the group because you don't feel you can join in, you're quite free to come back when you feel like it. I want you to relax. Nothing awful is going to happen'. Tom says 'what's the point, then?' Rose replies 'Well, that's what we're going to find out. You'll see!' She looks round. Everybody seems very anxious, Una and Vicky have alert smiles, the men look apprehensive. Dawn alone seems relaxed. Her attention is elsewhere. She does not seem to have heard anything Rose has said. Rose suggests that people should take turns to say their names. Dawn is still only half aware of what is going on, and has to have things explained to her. Vicky says 'she's not with it today, are you love?' Tom says his name is Marmaduke, which creases George. Encouraged by Rose people cross over the circle and introduce themselves to each other, shaking hands. Cyril gives Elsie a hug which surprises her (and everyone else). Rose suggests that people might like to find a partner: 'Choose anyone you like; the last person you said hello to, perhaps'. The group seem to find this surprisingly difficult. Dawn is taken aside by Vicky, and Tom goes over to Joan. After a moment Cyril and Elsie stand next to each other, leaving George and Una who grin at each other and take hands. As with Cyril's hug, this marks an important stage in the proceedings. Rose explains the process of mirroring whereby people follow each others movements (described on p. 79). Couples begin very slowly and tentatively but things begin to warm up as Rose calls for an increase in timing. People are told to exchange the role of leader for that of follower, and then, after a few minutes to reverse the process, moving other parts of their bodies as well as their hands and taking in the whole room instead of remaining in one place: 'it's easier if you concentrate on your partner's eyes and don't watch the parts that are moving'.

Some couples find more difficulty in all this than others. Dawn and Vicky are moving at half the speed of Joan and Tom; Una and George keep up a moderate pace but are obviously in harmony and enjoying themselves. Dawn suddenly stops. She is not protesting, but has simply decided that she has had enough of this. Rose signals to everyone else to stop too. They are to stay with their partners but do something different. In order to get to know their partner better they are going to perform a little experiment in seeing how observant they can be. First of all they are to look as closely as possible at the person they are with. What are they wearing? Next, one partner is to turn away while the other partner makes a small adjustment to his or her own appearance (a ring, a watch, a button, a tie, etc.). When he or she has done this, the other is to turn round. What has been changed? Now swap roles and do it again. It is at this point that the session begins to gain momentum. This is an easy game, and just personal enough to be enjoyable. (Having someone disturb their own clothing, even in so minor a way as not to cause embarrassment, can be a very friendly and reassuring gesture.) Rose is a bit concerned in case Tom abuses his privileged position as group member, but nothing untoward happens. Dawn seems to enjoy this part more than what went before. When it is her turn to change her appearance she becomes quite animated. She is delighted when Vicky doesn't notice that she is wearing one earring …

The process of getting to know each other carries on into the next stage of the session in which couples discuss a specially chosen topic of a controversial kind ('Should Prince Charles and Princess Diana send their children to a state school or a public school?'). All the couples have the same subject to argue about, but they certainly don't go about it in the same way. As with the mirroring exercise some work much faster than others. All the couples are busy talking, but Rose gets the impression they are all talking about something different. She moves round the room reminding them about the subject to be discussed. After a few minutes she warns everybody that their time is nearly up: will they draw their discussions to a close? A minute later she calls everyone into the centre of the room. Each person is asked to say what his or her partner has been saying. They do this *as if they were their partner*. For example, Cyril says, 'I am Elsie, and I think that we are very cheeky if we think we have any right to an opinion about what Prince Charles and Princess Diana decide to do about their own children. That's their affair!' Elsie, on the other hand, finds herself putting Cyril's more egalitarian views as if she had swapped identity and they were now her own. Tom seems to have missed the point, because he demands the right to speak for himself and keeps on butting in while Joan is pretending to be him. Rose patiently explains the rules once again. Tom grins. He will keep rules that suit him. He does not realise yet that he can actually make these rules work very much in his own favour; instead he thinks they are peculiar and rather eccentric.

The feeling in the group is much friendlier and more animated than it was to begin with. Rose comments on this, and several people nod in agreement. Elsie says 'yes, I've really enjoyed it'. Jean says 'it's been a bit funny, but it's made us know each other a bit better'. Rose says, 'Well, shall we see what we know about people in the group? Let's put people together who have something in common with each other'. People take turns at arranging the group according to any shared characteristics they can think of. It is done by getting people who are considered to be like each other in some way to stand together. People find this a bit difficult but seem to get the point. George puts Cyril, Elsie and Vicky next to one another 'because they are all kind people'. Dawn puts Vicky and Elsie together because she thinks both are like her mother. The other groupings are more mechanical (for instance Tom simply places all the women together). Perhaps this kind of process is too difficult at this stage, and requires more confidence than can be expected. It is enjoyed, however, and gives rise to a good deal of laughter. Rose reminds everybody that this place and time are to be a regular 'date' for everyone. She encourages people to say goodbye to one another, and particularly their partners. Elsie and Cyril hug again, followed this time by George and Una and Vicky and Dawn.

This was the first session for this group, and cohesion has not had time to develop yet. Some of the elements which will set it apart from the rest of life have begun to show themselves, mainly in and through the role-reversal exercises. Even Tom who threatened to be a source of disturbance had become more involved towards the end, as he found himself growing interested in what was going on. It will take time for him to value the occasion for what it has to offer him in terms of real self-expression and self-discovery rather than merely as an opportunity to show off in front of the women. On the other hand it is possible that Tom may never manage to identify completely with the group, in which case he will either leave it altogether or take up an ambiguous position, neither in the group nor out of it, acting as a narrator by commenting on whatever is going on. This is always a difficult situation to cope with, and every effort must be made to include such a person within the group. Members usually understand only too well what is going on, and co-operate in an effort to win such a person over. As for the rest of the group some imaginative links have been forged between individuals, and this is the first step in building up a viable group. At this stage personal development consists principally in overcoming a very natural nervousness. When we have a group, then we can start working with individuals; we shall also have to pay more attention to de-briefing.

Third session

The group meets in a large room in the Occupational Therapy Department of the Psychiatric Unit attached to a General Hospital. The room is divided at mid-point by folding doors. In the other half of the room patients are engaged in various kinds of art-work – pottery, weaving, basketmaking etc., so that there is a slight hum during every session from beyond the barrier. (The drama therapist has complained about this several times, but there is no other space available.) When Stephen, the drama therapist, arrives the group are already sitting in a circle. (He is not late; it is they who are early. This is because they are bored: They feel excluded from whatever is going on beyond the doors. There is an atmosphere of 'nothing ever happens here'.) There are only five people in the group – Christine, who is in her sixties, Jane and Yvonne, close friends, both around forty, Terry who is thirty-five but looks quite a lot younger, and Des, who is in his late teens. They know one another well and are the survivors of a group of twelve whom the drama therapist brought together almost a year ago. Mainly for social reasons these particular patients have remained in hospital. The therapist's main objective now is to prepare them for discharge. He is finding this difficult, because they intend to hang on to the bitter end.

When they see him they all exclaim with pleasure, moving up to make room for him in the circle. Terry lets go of Yvonne's hand. Jane takes hold of the therapist's: 'There!' The therapist is a bit taken aback at this. He doesn't want to be quite so cosy yet. With this group it might last the whole session! He says 'let's play a game, shall we?' Without much support, he sets about trying to interest the group in the game, making it up as he goes along. First of all, objects in the room are chosen in alphabetical order, and scattered around the room. The aim is to move as quickly as possible around each object in turn, without touching either the objects or one another. Each time an object is touched it is removed, and the speed of travel increased. People who touch are disqualified. The absurd nature of the improvised game has the desired effect and people are soon laughing and falling over one another. Yvonne says 'let's do it with our eyes closed.' This proves impossible because folk open their eyes every time they touch anything and can see to avoid the next obstacle. Christine suggests a way round the problem: people put their hands on the shoulders of the person in front and follow the leader, who has his or her eyes open. This works out better, and each member has a turn leading the group through the various hazards. When it is Stephen's turn he accompanies the journey with a commentary describing the kind of terrain through which they are passing. ('The night seems to be getting darker all the time – we're all right so long as we follow this line of fir-trees and keep walking on the smooth stones by the river. I think we're safer here by the river, but there's a lot of mud around, can you feel it?... My feet keep slipping off the stones, and so on'.)

The party finally arrive at a well in the middle of a wood. Each winds the bucket up. He or she is not to say what is reflected in the still water. Instead everyone is to open their eyes and return to their seats. Des says 'I should bloody well think so. You get carried away, Steve'. The leader begins to ask people what they saw reflected in the water. Yvonne says 'me, re-united with my loved ones'. Walking alone in the dark was 'becoming ill, not being loved and supported because of schizophrenia'. Yvonne has often mentioned missing her family, but this is the first time she has ever actually talked of her illness and the feelings she has about it – 'like walking along in the dark'. Christine says she saw her garden at home, 'not as it is now but as it could be'. She says that it made her feel guilty because it was so neglected 'like the way I let people down'. Terry says he saw 'a countryside of rich colours'. June says that she feels upset because she can't really get through the darkness – 'It's as if I'm still there as well as here. I'm on both sides of the barrier at once'. People talk about this, trying to get her to explain what she means. She can't do this; she has said what she means, and is pleased to have got it into words. Stephen turns to Des, expecting a bored response. 'I saw a pot of gold. I'm not kidding, I saw a great jar of gold reflected in the water'. People mull this over. Everyone seems impressed. After a pause, Stephen says, 'well, perhaps things may not turn out so badly after all'. He points out that the bad things that June and Christine have talked about were connected with the experience of walking through the dark rather than with the well, the past not the future. June begins to weep softly, and Yvonne puts her arms round her. Terry starts to talk about heaven – not jokingly but seriously. He doesn't get very far, perhaps because of a shortage of data. Everybody is somewhat subdued, but the atmosphere is considerably more relaxed than at the beginning of the session. Even Des is smiling, in a reflective way. Stephen says, quietly, 'They were your ideas, you know. I only took you on a journey'. Yvonne says 'it was what we did with the journey'. The group squeeze one another's hands. Stephen says 'we'll say thank you to one another, shall we?' They do this, before saying goodbye.

Looking back on this session the leader felt that there had been some degree of movement towards a positive view of leaving hospital. He had suggested an image of passing through difficulty into a kind of fulfilment, and they had all, to some extent, accepted this. Some of the imagery which surfaced combined hope and despair, which augured well for the prospect of learning how to carry pain without being totally defeated by it (Yvonne, June, Christine). All the group were familiar with the drama therapy approach and had no trouble adapting to the kinds of procedures involved, but this makes it all the more remarkable that their response was so fresh and unstereotyped. They were definitely bored to begin with, but this only lasted for a few minutes. Despite the rather unfavourable conditions the power of corporate imagination asserted itself; I don't think anybody noticed the hum from next door at all. There was a real feeling of coming to the surface again when it was all over. Admittedly the group knew one another rather well to begin with, so that they did not need time to adjust to being together. On the other hand they had shared interests and experiences which could have been very distracting if they had chosen to talk about them during the session. Instead they responded to the challenge of using their imagination creatively in the attempt to come to terms with the future.

Fourth session

The setting is a large sitting room in an Acute Ward of a psychiatric hospital. The building itself dates from the turn of the Century, but this ward has been up-graded and is reasonably bright and cheerful. The chairs have been pushed back against the walls, leaving a carpeted space in the centre of the room which measures roughly 20 by 20 feet. Jean is leading the group. She is a trained drama therapist. Her co-therapist, Grahame, is a nurse. The group has been meeting in this ward on a regular basis – twice a week for five months. Progress beyond a certain point is impeded by the fact that group members tend to come and go, in accordance with the admission policy of the hospital, and nobody stays for more than six or seven weeks at a time. At the moment the group consists of two elderly men (James and Richard), a middle-aged woman (Sophia), a man of around thirty-five (Peter), two young women in their mid-twenties (Gill and Steph) and a man of forty (Clive). This group has been together for a month, although James, Richard and Sophia have known one another for longer and James and Sophia were together in a previous group during their last stay in hospital.

When Jean and Grahame arrive, James and Richard are sitting next to the door, talking. None of the rest of the group is present. Looking round the room, Jean says to James 'It all looks a bit quiet today'. James says 'It's always quiet here'. Grahame has rounded up the rest of the group and managed to deflect them from the surrounding chairs so that they are standing roughly in a circle. Jean suggests a game 'to loosen us up a bit'. She produces a rubber ball; people are to say their own names and throw the ball to someone else. Gill and Clive put on bored expressions so that Jean wonders if she hasn't pitched the level too low – Clive's face says very clearly 'I'm an adult not a kid'. Gill is unwilling to relax because she doesn't want people – particularly Clive – to think her a fool. However, the game is quite hard to play properly because of the urge to say the other person's name instead of your own, and it becomes harder when another ball is introduced. Grahame congratulates Richard on his skill, and people get more interested. After a few minutes Steph says 'I'm feeling tired', and sits down on the carpet. Everybody does the same, relieved by the break in activity. 'It's a nice carpet', says Steph. 'Why don't we enjoy it more?' While preparing the session, Jean and Grahame have been thinking of an activity which would help people to trust one another more while at the same time stimulating their imaginations, so the group are encouraged to discover original ways of crossing the room, touching the carpet with as much, then as little, of themselves as they are able, crossing with a partner, or as a trio, then finally all together. This is welcomed as a good idea by the younger members, but after a few hilarious minutes, Richard and James have to be given permission to return to the chairs. (Richard is relieved at being 'let off the hook', and is a little put out by the fact that James is enjoying himself.)

Jean: 'I bet you could do it well enough once, Richard.'

Richard: 'You can say that again!' *(He is still rather put out).*

James: 'Come on, we've all got to get older.'

Richard: 'I could tell you. Just after I was married...'

James tries to quieten him, but he wants to tell the story. Jean has something else in mind, but she sees that the rest of the group are genuinely interested in hearing what Richard has to say. Having secured an audience, Richard describes an occasion 'many years ago' when he was mountain climbing in Wales and got lost in the mist. When the mist cleared he found himself on the very edge of a precipice. He could see the way down, but could not manage to get there because of a huge boulder blocking his way. With the help of a tree-trunk he dislodged the boulder, and got down the mountain in safety. 'I still dream about it sometimes. I get to the edge of the chasm and then I wake up.' Sophie says 'It's like a film.' 'It was worse than a film,' says Richard. After a slightly awe-struck pause, Clive says, very tentatively, 'shall we act it?' Jean asks Richard to go through the story again step by step. He is obviously pleased by the idea. Richard's chair is pulled into the centre of the carpet, and the rest of the group sit round him. The action of the drama is carefully plotted. It will have five scenes, 'getting lost', 'on the edge', 'overcoming the obstacle' (titles devised by Gill and Steph). Richard asks to be excused, at this point, from taking part: 'I don't want to go all through that again, thank you'. Steph tries to persuade him to have a go at it, but without success. Clive volunteers and is accepted by the group. Clive has lost the vague air of nervousness he had to begin with and seems much more confident. He says he will enjoy 'having a proper part to play'. Because there is only one real part, the rest of the group concentrate on providing Clive/Richard with an enthusiastically gregarious set of companions from whom to be separated. This part of the drama is much enjoyed by all, and particularly by Richard. It was Grahame's idea that the play should be presented 'in the round', with Richard's armchair in the centre of the circle, so that he should feel 'in the middle of things'. This means that Clive/Richard can wander round in a circle looking through the mist (represented by Sophia, Gill and Steph) – searching for the lost path. The precipice is directly in front of Richard's chair, and Clive/Richard must decide when to discover the full horror of his position. Just as he is about to do this, Richard leaves his chair and moves across to take up his position on the edge of the chasm. He pushes away Clive, who now becomes the boulder, joined first by Gill and Steph, then Peter, who soon decides he would rather be the crucial tree trunk and takes his stance alongside Richard. Richard and Peter shift the boulder.

This has been a considerable strain for everybody, with people pushing as hard as they were able. Everyone sits down again with relief. Richard, however, seems rather less tired than at the beginning of the session. We talk about the play. Jean says to Richard, 'So you found you could join in after all?' Richard says, 'I wanted to make sure you got it right'. Peter says 'it was fun'. Clive says 'perhaps you won't dream about it now'. Gill says 'he'll dream about our version instead!' There is a pause for a few seconds. Everybody smiles. People de-role by holding hands and saying one another's name. We arrange to meet again later in the week.

This was a session which moved away from its original intention which was to build cohesion and a sense of safety before any kind of personal exploration was embarked on. This seemed necessary because of the variations in age, group experience and psychiatric diagnosis. As it turned out there was a degree of trust in the group which made it possible to go further and deeper than we had expected, on the initiative of the members themselves. An interesting point about the session was the way in which the 'staging' of the drama corresponded to its subject matter and personal meaning. Certainly a world was created here in the imaginative involvement of the group. There was a very definite sense of the suspension of categories dividing people according to age, sex, physical and mental ability, class etc. The drama 'worked' because of this sharing of experience, which gave a strong impression of a new situation suggesting new rules. (This may also reflect the desire to escape from the actual setting even in imagination.) The quality of sharing was increased by the lack of overt direction – or directiveness – on the part of the leaders. It looked as though one of the group members, Peter, was not going to commit himself entirely to the session, but in the event he joined in fully, and the threatened 'narrator effect' did not occur. The atmosphere within the group was much happier at the end than the beginning. Clive (who had acted the principal role) seemed tired but peaceful. Richard, the real 'principal', was so far from his official anxiety-depression as to seem actually elated. Becoming aware of his body, with its aches and pains, had unlocked an imagination able to transcend them.

Case study

Tony's childhood was unextraordinary. He had been brought up in a Sheffield suburb during the years following the Second World War. Like so many others in the particular neighbourhood his social life was dominated by school and church. The school was the local Grammar School, and the church was Methodist. Tony's parents had decided not to send him to boarding school, although they could have afforded to do so. Instead they kept him at home, for much the same reason that they preferred the Methodist Church rather than the Parish Church. The family ethos centred around a kind of Puritanism. Protestant standards of morality were easier to maintain at home than away, and this went for religious practices as well. It was a family ethos that had been passed from generation to generation. Tony saw nothing wrong with it, despite the anguish involved in reconciling it – or rather failing to do so – with the emergent sexuality of adolescence. In the early 1960s Tony married a woman with a background similar to his own. The marriage was remarkably free from incident, Tony and Margaret dedicating themselves to preserving the traditional values of middle class family life and providing a secure background for their twin girls, for whose benefit the pattern of school and chapel was carefully repeated.

Round about the time of the children's sixteenth birthday, Tony's wife left him, and them, to live with a man she had met at a Chapel Anniversary dance. It was this domestic catastrophe that was considered to be the cause of the chronic anxiety states he developed over the next fifteen years. While the twins were at home he managed to perform adequately as a single parent, although the girls maintain that he was always exceedingly strict and allowed them very little freedom 'even though we were grown up'. This is probably why, as soon as they could manage it, they too left home.

When Tony first came to the Day Hospital, he was living by himself. One of the twins visited him twice a week. The other had gone abroad. Tony was diagnosed as suffering from anxiety-depression. He was a quiet self-deprecating person. At the level of ordinary social relationships he made friends easily enough, partly because of his eagerness to please, or at least, not to stand out as being awkward. When asked if he would be willing to join a drama therapy group, he said he had no objection. Why should he have? It was part of the treatment, after all.

Tony had reason to be grateful for having taken this attitude towards something which, in fact, made him rather nervous. In particular, Tony did not like the idea of exercises involving physical movement. He felt he had little grace and skill and had unhappy memories of school (he was rather overweight) and disliked being made self-conscious, which he certainly did not associate with any kind of psychiatric help he was able to imagine. As he said himself, 'we came here to get better, and you're making us all feel worse'. He was only partly joking. As a matter of fact the remark was more constructive than he knew, formulating an attitude which bound the group together, helping them to overcome their individual uncertainties. It also demonstrated that one could 'be oneself' and still remain within the group, which was the most important thing of all. As drama therapy is built upon movement, Tony had plenty of opportunity to get used to the feel of his own body, something he had never before been encouraged to do. Sessions often begin with some kind of exploration of our physical experience. On one occasion, vital for Tony's restoration to health, the group were walking about imagining that the floor was a sea shore covered in warm dry sand. People were encouraged to kick their feet through the sand, let it run through their toes, bury their heels in it as deeply as they could lifting their toes in the air, run across it, sit down on it, do handstands etc. Next, they were to imagine the sand had changed to something else. The same kinds of things were to be done, but the medium was now quite different. After a few minutes, Tony left the room. He didn't come back until the session was nearly over. People were talking about a mime they had been working on; when Tony started to talk about the sand they were not really interested. The Leader, sensing that here was something Tony really wanted to share with the group, asked him what his special material had been.

Tony: It felt like ground glass. It didn't hurt, though. You could kick your feet in it as if it were sand. It was strange, though.

Leader: How? Can you tell us?

Tony: It's a bit silly, really.

Geoff *(group member):* That's all right, isn't it? *(He secures the attention of the rest of the group).*

Tony: The ground glass kept getting clear. Every second or third step it became like a window and you could see things.

Pat *(group member):*   What sort of things? *(A pause)*

Tony: Don't laugh. *(He is visibly shaken).*

Leader: Nobody's going to laugh. It was your experience. You tell us.

Tony: Beasts. Monsters.

Geoff: You mean like a horror movie?

Tony: No, real monsters. But like kid's monsters. There's a book, *Where the Wild Things Are.* Like that. I knew these things; they were horrible...

Tony was willing to let some of the monsters be presented in mime. He would not take part in this himself, but gave graphic instructions to the group as to size, appearance, ways of moving etc. (He even had definite ideas about noise and smell.) As the session proceeded Tony became more involved in what was going on. He never became a 'wild thing' himself, but when the menagerie was complete he took his place in the centre of the action as if he were ring master. The creatures began to dance round him making hideous noises. For a moment it was very frightening indeed. Afterwards Tony said he had been terrified. He kept his hands close in at his sides, holding on to the seams of his trousers. Then, suddenly, he lifted his hands over his head and laughed aloud.

When everyone had had enough stomping and shrieking, people subsided to the floor.

Tony: I'm sorry. *(Pause)*

Philip *(group member):*   We enjoyed it.

Leader: How are you feeling?

Tony: I've got a headache. I don't want to say anything.

Mary *(group member):*   It was fun. Thanks, Tony. Can I ask you just one thing? Did you *recognize* anyone?

Tony: Oh, yes.

Leader: Perhaps Tony would like to talk, but not yet. Is that right, Tony?

Tony: I don't know. Yes. Not yet.

Mary: Well, it was a game. We made it up, didn't we?

Soon afterwards the session ended, members making sure that Tony wasn't by himself. The next session was largely led by Tony who wanted to explore the monsters again and relate them to things about himself and other people. He said he felt better: 'better than I've felt for a long time. Much less anxious'.

This episode illustrates some of the most important things about the medium. Most obviously it is an example of the function of drama therapy as an aid to *self-disclosure*. As Dorothy Langley has succinctly stated: 'In this way we see that acting is not a matter of donning a mask and pretending, but of removing a mask and revealing' (1983: 102). Kicking your feet through imaginary sand may be just as effective a way of removing your mask as playing Hamlet is. It is certainly a *bodily state* involving the release of nervous tension. It is *active* rather than passive, concerned with experiencing the world in an immediate way (at ground level, perhaps!) It happened within a special kind of social setting providing the essential *structure* for therapeutic encounter and imaginative involvement. This could not have taken place without the complete understanding and acceptance of the group and the sense of corporate identity which gave courage to each individual member. A special place, a special time; at this point in Tony's life past, present and future coincided in an experience of *insight* able to make sense of an entire personal history: to make it a history rather than the mere succession of events.

This is the real purpose of the medium, to present us with a metaphor of life, and so to direct attention to the meaning of the things that happen to us. The structure which we crave is implicit in the metaphor. We do not find our personal metaphor easily. It is hard to appreciate the outline of even that part of the forest we know well. When we climb a tree we can see very little apart from more trees, and the unfathomable sky. We need some way of lifting ourselves up above the place we know so we may catch a glimpse of what the forest really is, where it stretches from and reaches to. We all need this, but some are more claustrophobic than others.

These drama therapy sessions have been chosen for description because they are more or less typical of the rather low-key dramas in which almost everybody finds themselves involved in the course of ordinary living – scenarios about the significant events in which we are involved, and about our own self image, as we see ourselves in the eyes of other people. Despite its name, the actual content of drama therapy is not often dramatic. However, the disclosures to which it gives birth can sometimes be very significant.

Notes

1. The inventor of psychodrama had little time for the kind of psychotherapy which measured success in terms of an irreducible increment of predictable behavioural change, taking place in the direction of a rigidly stereotyped definition of what may be taken to constitute 'mental health' or 'social adjustment'. Moreno was quite sure that healing can only partially depend on general notions and must vitally concern each individual's own evaluation. 'Validation in individual and group psychotherapeutic practice is not imperative, so long as no pretence is made that generalisations can

be drawn from whatever the events recorded or that the future behaviour of the participants can be predicted from the events. What matters is that the therapeutic experiences are valid for the participants themselves, at the time they take place' (1972: 216).

2. 'Qualitative procedures...reject the assumption that objectivity can only be secured through quantitative or scientific methods... Let the problem determine the method, not vice versa' (1985: 136).

Chapter 8

Drama Therapy and Ritual

Trying life out for size, gauging the personal meaning of different ways of behaving, belongs to the very basis of being human. In this book I have examined, briefly and inadequately, some of the ways that an understanding of the nature and significance of drama can help us to understand more about, and consequently do more to relieve, particular psychoses. In the final chapter, the scope is widened. I have suggested that both drama and psychotherapy owe their ability to heal to something else. This 'something else' is considerably easier to describe than to explain, if indeed one should want to explain it. Its most striking manifestations are to be found elsewhere, away from the psychiatric clinic and the extemporised drama session, in the heightened atmosphere and vividly intensified experience of religious ritual and certain kinds of theatre – theatre at its most self-conscious and least naturalistic, concerned with life's metaphysical implications, not its outward appearance. Chapter 1 concerned the theatrical foundations of drama therapy. This chapter returns to the theme of drama therapy's strong links with religious ritual, which is able to give it another dimension, one that is exceedingly important, and without which it cannot really be understood.

Because it explores the relationship of persons, theatre's attention is always to some extent directed towards the meaning of life. The approach is characteristically oblique: not thrusting its message at us, but allowing us to make contact in our own way, at our own speed. Meetings of this kind are open to the God who moves between, whether those involved hold any specific faith or none. Secular involvement in drama owes its inspiration to an urge to discover meaning in the relationship of persons and the story of interpersonal events which gives rise to particular religious systems. Historically, drama, religion and healing all spring from the same source. Because meaning develops in line with human experience, growing and changing in accordance with the urge to arrange and re-arrange events so that they will provide support for our own particular 'construct systems', life is thought about in terms of story, a series of associated events reaching a particular conclusion. This may be final, drawn by others when we die; or it may be provisional, as we ourselves stand back and take stock of what has happened, is happening now, even while we are thinking about it. In a story, events speak louder than words, in the sense that the preferred mode of communication is narrative rather than exposition. Many details can be left unexplored so long as the story itself 'holds together'. Each story has a 'point'. This may not be obvious, but it is always there. Otherwise it is not a story. Stories offer us the chance of an alternative world. We may, or may not, choose to take up the offer, but it has been made. Sometimes it is particularly hard to resist, as some worlds exert a powerful magnetism. A million such worlds exist, thousands within our own culture, ranging from the Forest of Arden to the 'island full of noises', from Erewhon to Middle Earth, taking in Narnia and a complete genre of 'fantasy fiction' on the way. Some of these are creations which possess a resonance eluding analysis, striking at the heart of a profounder awareness than the conscious one. The story itself does not create this awareness but directs our attention powerfully towards it. Wherever there is an element of story the symbolic effect occurs. We experience people and events that are islanded from immediate reality, separated from the rest of life by an ocean of selective remembering and forgetting, a simplified world of pure signification.[1]

This world, free from distraction and irrelevance, is the dimension in which we encounter the profoundest truth about ourselves. Wherever men and women journey through life together, a story emerges to give the idea reality. The religious awareness of many peoples takes mental shape as a narrative, lending itself to dramatic representation. Stories of heroes and heroines, saviour figures, saints and sinners, builders of community and rebels against an unwelcome order, past epiphanies and future apotheoses: in all these story produces drama, and drama embodies faith. The history of drama makes this fact obvious. In Classical Greece, for instance, the drama actually originated in the cultus, emerging from the religious dances, the dirges and incantations which were supposed to have a curative effect, promote immortality or fertility, or ensure victory in battle. The therapeutic use of drama was very close to its religious nature, therapeutic drama having its roots in early healing rituals in which movement and incantation uniting body, mind and spirit were known to have a curative effect involving the experience of total personal communication. Indeed, students of classical Greek culture are accustomed to attribute responsibility for the birth of the Western theatrical tradition to the yearly festivals which took place at various shrines through the Mediterranean world, and particularly those which were held in celebration of Dionysus, god of life and death, who was believed to have been torn apart and yet to have survived. Out of the rites associated with Dionysus, at some time during the 6th Century BC, there began to emerge the most primitive form of stage play. This was based on the elaborate choral performance of the dithyrambs, hymns dedicated to the dying and rising god, which described the incidents in his life among men. Thus dramatic dialogue is, in historical terms, the expansion and articulation of a healing narrative.[2]

Examples of the ritual origin of theatre are to be found in the well established theatrical traditions of other cultures. Classical theatre in India and Japan is also clearly religious in origin. The Indian drama has its roots in the Vedas, the oldest and most sacred of the Indian scriptures. Hindus believe that Brahma, the creative principle of the universe, invented the drama as a precious source of spiritual fulfilment and simple pleasure, to be enjoyed equally by men and by the gods. Dancing was introduced into dramatic performances by Shiva, Lord of time, death, and the destruction of appearances, to broaden the scope of the plays' subject-matter and produce emotional and intellectual verisimilitude. Vishnu, the Hindu principle of continuity and ongoing development, divided the new artistic creation into the four styles of classical Hindu drama, each one separate from, and yet closely related to, the others.[3]

Similarly, one of the main sources of the Japanese Noh tradition was the pageantry associated with shrines at festival times. The great medieval dramatist Zeami Motikoyo taught that an actor should dedicate his life to the Noh with the very greatest personal devotion, using spiritual exercises to prepare for what was in fact a religious celebration. Noh plays were originally presented in cycles of five dramas, with farcical interludes interspersed among them. The spirit of a religious devotion to the art of presenting truth in dramatic form imbued the entire series, which was regarded as a corporate experience of healing rather than an acted sermon. There is a fundamental similarity between the Noh plays and the Medieval Mysteries; basically, despite obvious cultural differences, they were the same kind of theatre.

The tradition remains, affecting the way we regard theatre even today. Peter Brook says that 'the notion that the stage is a place where the invisible can appear has a deep hold upon our thoughts' (1968). I would go further and say that theatre, and the dramatic action in which it originates, is where we *make* invisible things visible. For all concerned, theatre is active, not passive. This is true of the back row of the gallery as well as the front row of the stalls. Always, and everywhere, the healing power of theatre abides in participation, in action as well as passion, giving as well as taking. The things we see, hear, understand and interiorise, use and reject, are things we have contributed, our own things as well as things that we have made our own. Here, as in all our life the healing power of the human spirit lies in its ability to share and be shared. Through the instrumentality of the dramatic idea, this instinct of love – for that is what it is – is focused and magnified, so that it may become strong enough to pierce the clouds around our heart and kindle the fire which is ready to leap into flame in celebration of the most important thing about us – that we are human and that we *care*.

This is the 'irrational living force' that Artaud warns us about: a presence barely held in check by our judgements as to what is sensible, or socially acceptable, or in line with our own personal way of looking at life. Drama is able to make this presence active within us, to unchain its forces and set them to work upon our lives. It can be 'cruel' because of the effect it has on our own selfishness, the gaping breach it makes in walls painstakingly erected and scrupulously reinforced over many years. We did not know we had feelings like these, having spent so much effort not to know, or at least not to acknowledge their full intensity. Now we feel their biting edge, and are amazed at ourselves.

The feelings come, of course, from the drama's original identity, the ritual stories of the gods, whose theme is nothing less than the religious journey of mankind, healing of the spirit expressed in narrative form. Thus it is story that provides the link between spirituality and drama therapy, expressing itself in scenarios of personal and corporate change which take the form of journeys, ascents, crossings, voyages, penetrations, arrivals and departures, passages of all kinds. In shamanistic rituals, the priest or shaman leads his disciples on a journey in which he and they undergo experiences of a growing intensity, leading them out of the world of prosaic events, the ordinary life of everyday, into a place and time which is unrecognisable, where pain and pleasure, sense and nonsense, images of living and dying, are first intensified and then transformed. A place which is no place, because none of the familiar landmarks exist and our ordinary ways of coping with what happens to us, the familiar sense we make of life, has lost its usefulness. The things learned in this central condition, it is claimed, may not be guessed in advance. They have not happened yet. Their relevance belongs to the Journey home, the third stage of the shamanistic experience, in which life is lived in a new way, in the light of what has been learned en route.

Thus, throughout the world, religious rituals assert the difference between earth and heaven, allowing believers to step from one reality to another, strengthened in being by experiencing the carefully contrived contrast between them. Everywhere, the shape of the journey is that of the rite of passage, the three-fold ritual complex embodying change and growth by means of an actual voyage from place to place. In such rites the crucial central stage, the 'time-out-of-time' in which change occurs, is symbolised by a geo-graphical location – a desert or forest to cross, a mountain to climb, caves which we must penetrate in order to be re-born.

Ritual precedes theatre both developmentally and with regard to its closeness to the source from which both draw their life, which is the human urge to refresh oneself at the source of personal life, however this may be intellectually understood, if it is intellectually understood at all. It is a tightening and intensification of our inter-personal awareness which uses the dramatic mode which is our natural way of expressing ourselves in a special way, by changing the social convention from the one used for the everyday exchanges of commerce, leisure, education, family life, intimate personal relations to one specially reserved for dealing with ultimate concerns and final meanings. In ritual we get down to truth in a way we find difficult elsewhere. Nothing interrupts us here; what goes on refers to ordinary life, but is not entirely governed by it. A salutary shift of our frame of reference keeps us from being distracted by what is happening 'outside'.

If drama demonstrates how we normally relate to one another, ritual shows us how to relate to values that are ultimate. The social bond is, to use Goffman's terminology,[4] 'purer' than it is in theatre; those involved are caught up within a single action, the expression of a mutually accepted intention. Ritual has no audience – aesthetic distance is located between worshipped and worshippers, whatever the object of worship may be, and those involved are drawn together by a shared action. The brackets that we erect round corporate rituals, signifying a change of social convention necessitating a new kind of understanding and relating are more clearly marked than they are in theatre, where they are largely played out for us, and require submission rather than conscious co-operation.

The result is a happening of considerable toughness and resilience, one which is able to survive in the least promising circumstances and with only a few people taking part. Indeed, the value of a rite is not usually deemed to depend so much upon the way that it is performed as is the case with plays. All the same, it is necessary to pause for a second before even the most unassuming public ritual in order to 'change gear', whereas it may be possible to 'go straight into' a piece of drama, thereby increasing the realism. Ritual is scarcely interested in realism. (It is interesting to see how theatre grows more ritualistic as the events it portrays become more extraordinary. Macbeth is a case in point).

The formal characteristics of ritual are all-important. It communicates mainly by its shape – the inescapable clarity of beginning, middle and end. The structures of the rite are simpler and the order with which they proceed clearer than in the theatre. There is a greater concentration on *experiencing* than *explaining*. Ritual stands by itself, contributing as much to society and to individuals as it demands from them in the way of involvement in its action and devotion to its purpose. Precisely because it is less real than ordinary social life, less beguiling than the naturalistic dramas we play out every day among ourselves, it has a greater hold on our attention.

Drama therapy shares important formal similarities with religious ritual. Both drama therapy and corporate ritual are ways of implementing interior change, in that they have regard to the actual shape of the events, interior and exterior, which symbolise the reality of such changes. By drawing closer to the source of being itself, the power that lives between and among persons, we are strengthened and enriched. We move onwards in living and upwards in being. To this extent, every ritual, whether secular or religious, that involves the meeting of persons, is a rite of passage.

Ritual change takes place in three stages, according to which a threshold of human experience is approached, crossed, and passed, in the sense of being achieved. The actual moment of change is treasured for intensity rather than extent. It has to be prepared for and taken account of. Unless it is taken seriously, it will not happen as a real event. Because it involves leaving the past behind as the sole condition of movement into the future, it is hard to encompass. Our involvement with what we know already, the way we are now, is the measure of the harshness of our experience of discontinuity, which characterizes the crossing of the threshold. Without an intervening period of disorientation, however, no real change can take place. Before new life can be established, old life must have already died. The three-fold rite reproduces the shape of human transformation, by underlining the 'time-between' which holds past and future apart. Real changes always happen like this. There is always a time of adjustment[5] which necessitates a kind of dying to what has gone before. The rite explores this 'fact of life', when the future is severed from the past by an experience of discontinuity which is always disturbing and often frightening, partly because we are so unwilling to explore it on our own, preferring to move directly between two ways of living, as if such a thing were possible. We have seen how, by concentrating on the autonomy of the first and last stages of a drama therapy session, the therapist is able to create a central space in which change may take place. The order of events within the session itself suggests personal change, the 'passage of the magical threshold which is a transit into a sphere of rebirth'.[6] Here, as in the rite of passage the protected central area is spatial as well as temporal. Here, however simply, some version of a myth of salvation is re-enacted and we break through into a richer life. The mixture of danger and safety, so fundamental to drama therapy, corresponds to the 'pivoting of symbolism' which makes embarkation upon a spiritual voyage both attractive and terrifying. We want to be both liberated from and confirmed in our present way of being. Our only hope lies in our reaching beyond, yet how shall we survive without the familiar evidence, the tried and tested formulae?

Neither drama therapy nor religious ritual make compromises. Both set out to tighten our hold upon 'ordinary' reality, before they launch us into that which is radically different. The state of mind which allows us to move creatively away from our present truth into an unknown truth of the future rests on a sureness of who we are in the here and now, a 'tightening' of our 'personal construct system' corresponding to the celebration of group identity which takes place in the preliminal rite and the first third of a drama therapy session. After this, constructs are 'loosened' and the possibility of newness is disclosed.

In such a context newness and healing belong together. The ability to receive spiritual healing is limited by the ability to conceive wherein healing consists. In order to grow as people we must have constructs of self-transcendence; that is, we must have developed a system of anticipating events which is able to take increasingly greater risks in reaching out for things guessed at, hoped for, but not yet properly understood. The whole enterprise of drama therapy is a way of helping individual women and men past the horizons which limit them, into ever expanding spheres of personhood.

Helping them past. The use of symbolism is crucial. Jung has described how symbols filter the healing experience of spirit, while protecting us from direct encounter with truths that are more than we can cope with in our present condition.[7] The drama therapy space connects two kinds of reality, acting like that meeting place between earth and heaven which Eliade identifies as an original religious symbol – the tree of heaven, the navel of the created universe which is the place of birth and re-birth (1958, Chs. 10–12). This is the arena of myth, in which our life takes on a significance larger than itself. In rites of passage the mythic hero is conceived of as departing from this spot, to realize his destiny. His adult deeds, says Campbell, 'pour creative power into the world'. This heroic action is 'a continuous shattering of the crystallizations of the moment' (1988: 337). The heart of the ritual-dramatic encounter is a 'microscopic mirror of the macrocosm'.

Thus drama therapy and ritual help us make sense of ourselves by making sense of our relationship with others and with the cosmos. The latter gives transcendental validity to the former. In cultures which retain an acknowledged religious social identity, society is made visible to itself as participating in the godhead by means of such rituals. Individual members of such societies find that their vision is enlarged by ritual identification with the hero of the rite, who is not limited by past, present or future circumstance; who, though he suffers, always triumphs. The *katharsis* of ritual is the archetype of that redemption of private self-preoccupation by identification with another's pain on which dramatic *katharsis* depends. In the rite of passage, it corresponds to the transformation of personal and social life brought about by nature's involvement with the hero's dying and surviving. The assurance of new life is explicit – Campbell calls such rituals 'grace-yielding sacraments' (1988: 23). So is the evidence in favour of drama as a therapeutic medium.

Whether it be in ritual or drama, such a cathartic experience depends on a particular relationship of *dramatis personae*. What happens is as important as to whom it happens. The stories which express and embody religious belief throughout the world correspond to the story-telling which plays such an important part in drama therapy.[8] In religious myth, someone voyages away from the place he knows into the unknown; there he carries out an adventure, or simply remains in hardship or danger of some kind; finally, he or she returns and the event is received as a deliverance. This is the archetypal form of the myth, a story which conducts us away from our habitual frames of reference, loosening our construct systems and breaking down the fixed patterns of neurotic thinking with the permeability of the symbolic narrative. To allow oneself to enter the sphere of myth is to travel along a path which has the fragility of a dream and the rock-like endurability of the dream's real meaning – the meaning that underlies and sustains life itself, and which can be experienced but not analysed. The experience of such meanings transforms our relationship to life and death.

Thus myth transmits a message about divine order and wholeness existing in relationship to the 'changes and chances' of life in this world. Myth and rite belong together, insofar as it is the interaction of a story and the rite which embodies and extends it that creates the myth. The historical precedence of rite over myth, or vice versa, has long been a matter of contention among historians of religion. The experience of drama therapists suggests that myth evolves from ritual. Stories are articulated by rites of passage designed to give them metaphorical significance by establishing pivotal points marking changes of direction in the journey of the hero. In this way, myths are created out of the lived imagination of the community as this is hammered out on the anvil of ritual. The shape of the hero's journey corresponds to the 'deeply significant motifs of the perils, obstacles and good fortunes of the way'...which form 'the everlastingly recurrent themes of the wonderful song of the soul's high adventure'.[9] This is the song of experience, not of wish-fulfilment. It is however experience of a particular kind – the paradoxical safety-out-of-danger symbolised in the rite of passage.

Drama therapy does not confine itself to a particular myth, but rather makes use of the ritual mechanisms which underlie mythological systems, the deepening and focusing of experience and the living-out of shared imagination. Certain mythic themes recur from time to time. For instance it is hard to progress as a drama therapy group without using some kind of 'heroic journey' mythology. The symbols which emerge are of a religious kind, even though none of the individuals involved lays claim to any kind of religious belonging. This is not surprising, of course – the imagery of the search for some kind of 'final meaning' is bound almost by definition to resemble that of religion. Not only this, but the use of art to express and explore experience is a proper way of getting into contact with spiritual truth at the deepest level of awareness. This is the kind of symbolism that Jung called 'the God within' (1938: 72). It is not surprising that it seems so much like a rite of passage.

As drama therapists we use the language of ritual because it suits our purposes so well, being, as it is, the dramatic expression of fundamental experiences of wholeness. Ritual says things we cannot say any other way. It can be primitive and powerful, yet capable of the utmost subtlety of meaning. Its language is self-explanatory, once we have invented it. Faced with new kinds of reality, we improvise ways of looking at them in their own terms. Just as mathematicians cannot adequately transmit information about mathematical relations without resorting to their own language of number, so we ourselves cannot describe reality without pointing out that what is merely talked about is quite precisely not what is actually being experienced. It is brought home to us that the language of ritual is actually its own truth. It is not a commentary upon, *or even a metaphor for*, anything else which might be considered to logically precede or metaphysically transcend it.[10]

We use it because it is the native tongue of mysteries too profound to be described in words, which are the general medium in which we work. Knowing too well the inadequacy of words to express our deepest longings for serenity and fulfilment, for healing of personhood, we are grateful for ritual. George Steiner has reminded us of the unreliability of words when it comes to describing the things that really matter to us: 'Words distort: eloquent words distort absolutely'. Ritual does not depend on words but on the transforming actions of lived life, the factual articulations which constitute a real event. Thus when drama therapy deals with the fundamental longings of the human soul, it speaks the language of religion, even though nothing 'religious' is actually said.

When it does this it goes a little way towards satisfying a great longing in the heart of man and womankind. We have few such rituals left, and almost none that are available to people who do not belong to a particular religion. Because of an instinctive desire to recognise landmarks or milestones in the lives by some kind of symbolic gesture carried out in public, and concerning a definitive metaphysical presence, whether it be human or divine in origin, most Western people are only 'religious' when they attend baptisms, weddings or funerals, the few remaining rites of passage we possess. The clergy look on grudgingly, wondering why their church should suddenly have become so attractive. It must be the opportunity the occasion presents to make a splash and impress the neighbours. This is not the only reason, however. In the presence of sacramental ritual there is a suspension of distrust. It is the church's words which puzzle and inhibit people, the things it says as 'the church', even though we know it is only the Vicar, or the Parish Priest, saying them. People come for the things that are *done* – the splashing, the bonding, the anointing, the taking-breaking-sharing of bread – the unambiguous expression of intention, of a world changed by the intending. It is as if we have a longing for the historical gestures of ritual.

In fact, these gestures are made historical, given a metaphysical significance, by the way in which they are presented, which in turn depends on the personal involvement of the presenters, their commitment to preserving the clarity of the message. It is exactly the same thing with regard to drama therapy, which cannot simply be seen as a series of techniques to be used pragmatically as the occasion may seem to suggest. Many things have to be taken into consideration before we launch 'spontaneously' into an alfresco session. In some way, perhaps unspoken, never completely unnoticed, the drama therapeutic process will work if given the chance to do so, so that there will be a proper beginning, middle and end, corresponding to the shape of a perfect event, the pre-liminal, liminal and post-liminal rituals of the rite of passage. Those involved must be fully aware of what is going to happen and the convention governing their own involvement in it. Interpersonal reality must be as mutual as possible, and arranged in ways that everybody understands. In other words, drama therapists must learn to build their own church if they want to celebrate the liturgy of persons as it should be celebrated.

We have seen how drama therapy is able to experiment with a range of different modes of presenting interpersonal reality in order to develop a flexible view of life in those taking part, increasing their versatility for dealing with the subtle shifts that occur in the conventions which govern our perception of the present moment. No theatre can play things quite like this; to present the action to an audience there must be some kind of unanimity. Events have to take place serially and according to one theatrical convention at a time, or tragedy will cancel comedy and romance be made ridiculous by farce. Playing to itself, drama therapy is in the position to tell counterpoint from confusion. This abundance of human experience, which is the celebration of life as it is, is the legacy of theatre, and when the drama therapeutic process involves confrontation, struggle and resolution, it must thank theatre for the ensuing *katharsis*.

Drama therapy needs both ritual and theatre. Separated from its roots, it degenerates into an exercise in role imitation undertaken for purposes of education or training, with no power to reach us at the level at which our experience of the world is changed. Without the inspiration of ritual and the imagination of drama it is no more than any other group therapy, with no unique contribution to make to the healing of persons.

As it is, drama therapy plays a unique part in psychotherapy. Here relationship as a public event, the experience of theatre, falls into line with relationship at its most intimate, the primal meeting of persons. Healing, like Spirit, moves among and between us; each member of the group 'bears the other's burdens', helped to do this by the dramatic structure, which allows the sharing of pain in *katharsis*. Problems and difficulties outside the group and within it are distanced by being presented in imaginative form, so that they can be lived rather than simply thought about – another form of burden-bearing which has distinctly religious overtones. In the living presence of the group, ideas and objects become imbued with a special personal significance, leading members into an ever closer relationship as they are invested with a kind of metaphysical power. This is the sign of focused meaning or intensified regard, the symbol of a love that is shared, expressing the group spirit. It may be centred on an object, a phrase, or a person. It speaks of and for the group, just as the group itself speaks of and for fellowship and communion. This is the group as 'transitional object', based in drama and play, the use of imagination, yet feeling unmistakably religious.

We have seen that two major distortions of human experience are affected positively by drama therapy's skill in the manipulation of structure to establish aesthetic distance. A personal world which is felt to be too present, and one which is too absent, are brought into a more tolerable balance by the experience of relationship mediated by drama therapy. Depression and schizophrenia are major psychoses. The special world which the drama creates, whose reality is contingent and yet in some ways convincing, allows a degree of experimentation, safe experimentation, in alternative ways of interpreting the evidence about oneself and other people; the ritual power of drama therapy is somehow able to incorporate the results of these experiments within the self. The psychologically loosening effect of drama is well established. That it should contain properties of structure able to tighten the 'loose' construct systems of people suffering from thought disorder is at first more surprising. It makes very little sense until we remember that theatre makes its own rules, and ritual makes them stick. The rules of theatre are clear but not binding (not outside the theatre, at least). They are easily distinguished, conveying the same message to everyone present, brought home to the audience as part of an inclusive, if temporary, reality. In the theatre everything contributes to the final impression, making a kind of focused sense, a conclusion which must be obvious even to someone who has been mystified and confused by life so that he or she can no longer 'think straight'. This is not true of all plays, or all productions of any one play, but it is the aspect of drama incorporated in drama therapy and realized in people's lives by the power of the rite. Along with it is the obvious demonstration of human contingency, as alternative ways of behaving, alternative ways of being, come to life within the scene. In drama therapy, a depressed person has the opportunity to change roles him or herself, and experience the reality of the changed feelings and attitudes that emerge when you ally yourself with another kind of personality living a different life from the one which is such a burden. Drama therapy aims at creating a new world for new things to happen in.

At this time there is a movement in drama therapy to re-discover its roots. These are not seen in psychotherapy, or even in psychodrama, but in theatre and in ritual. The recently formed Institute of Dramatherapy has strong links with the theatre, and organizes a yearly Shakespeare Seminar, taking place in Stratford-upon-Avon and involving workshops and discussions with members of the Royal Shakespeare Company. A growing number of dramatherapists have worked in the theatre, some with directors of international reputation, such as Joan Littlewood, Peter Brooke and Jerzy Grotowski. Members of staff at the Royal Academy of Dramatic Art 'double' as instructors on the Institute's Diploma Course in Dramatherapy, while experimental theatre is included as part of the training at four other centres where students are taught drama therapy at a post-graduate level.

So long as Sue Jennings has been associated with drama therapy – which is from the beginning – it has had a strong anthropological bias. This continues to be the case. During the last few years, Christian liturgiologists have begun to show interest, seeing how much ground they have in common with the actors and directors.[11] Psychotherapists and psychiatrists have always given support, fascinated by a less clinical approach to human problems than the usual ones. Now they are playing a more active part.

In fact, all sorts of people are exploring the possibilities of drama therapy. Some remain on the edges, attending an occasional day workshop, using a 'drama therapy approach' to smooth away obstacles between members of groups which they are 'running'. This attitude annoys people who take the approach seriously, having glimpsed its fascination as a philosophy of healing which is different from any other. The distinguishing characteristic of drama therapy is not its underlying psychopathology, which tends towards eclecticism, or its technical armamentarium, which it may share with psychotherapies such as Psychodrama and Gestalt; the unique property of drama therapy is its use of imagination. This alone puts it above approaches which recognise fantasy only in order to translate it into something else, something which may be included with the rest of common reality as a symptom or a complex of something quite well known. For drama therapy the imagination is the raw material of a transformed reality, working at the foundations of human experience, the truths about ourselves which are known but not understood, and are glimpsed only dimly in a world made up of a combination of common sense and specialisation. This is imagination about the meaning of life and death, an exploration of the happenings that take place on our journey 'from cradle to grave', the relationships which make the journey real to us. There is no question here of aligning particular problems with ready-made solutions. Instead, heaven is sung and the earth danced, the road followed to wherever it leads, past, present or future, only on this road everything is future, because everything is *possibility*. It is a matter of myth not science, as moods and memories are evoked which are able in their own strange way to convince us of continuity and consequently of purpose. Thus, shamanistic movements and gestures embodying the range of human attitudes to life and the natural world – powerful, flowing movements of control and mastery, abrupt staccato impositions of will, silent immobility and rest within the circling universe; the chaos of the unformed and uncontrolled in which the past has died and there is no future yet; the birth of beauty and love, in which meaning is discovered – stamp in us an awareness of participation in life and our own relevance to it. It is our world, and we can change it, but only by drawing close and rediscovering our place in it...

Such experiences bring home the interdependence of the spiritual and the physical, ideas and presences, the human and the divine. The process is one of reconciliation of body and mind, as though, by passing through an experience of dissolution they re-discover each other once more and the universe falls back into shape. Humanly speaking, it is on imagination alone that this kind of experiential transformation depends; but it is imagination made flesh, creating a new world to be incorporated within the life story of an individual and a group.

The events and disclosures, about people, times and places, owe their realism to the power of drama to convince us that such and such a thing is really happening. On the other hand, their ability to change us is an act of will, more to do with the quality of conviction which ritual carries with it, a definite choice rather than a surrender, however willing. In this kind of ritual drama therapy, you are present *as yourself*, not via identification with a 'character' in a play. In all drama therapy there must be a general willingness to 'believe in' what is going on and temporarily ignore the comments of the spectator-self as irrelevant to the meaning and purpose of the exercise. This kind of drama therapy demands a more profound involvement, a greater degree of concentration; perhaps even an element of self-sacrifice, as those taking part come to realize that letting go of one's present self, abandoning a cherished role, putting one's self-image at risk, re-opening old wounds, reliving past failures, will be painful if it is done properly. To allow it to be done at all, there has to be commitment to the enterprise. At this level, drama therapy carries the conviction that the search for ultimate truth bestows on those involved in it. It makes demands on its clients which are just as onerous as those made by any other kind of psychotherapy. But they are of a different kind and promise a different kind of reward.

This final chapter has concentrated on the idea of drama therapy as a spiritual search. This has led us into areas of life which seem to be a good deal removed from what might perhaps be considered a more rational approach. It should be remembered, however, that while the processes that have been described here cannot be analysed, the effects of living through them can sometimes be measured. There seems to be little doubt that such incursions into mystery may have the effect of clarifying rather than confusing the mind. These shared adventures into other worlds loosen the tight knots in our ways of construing reality, so that we are able to re-order our ideas and feelings and free ourselves for new ways of relating to people and events in the future. The deeper the initial mystery, the greater the final clarity. Just as the experience of relationship in drama results in a renewal of perceptual and cognitive structuring, so the actual shape of the dramatic journey creates and defines the futures to which it leads. We may have little religious faith or none at all. If we have a sense of mystery and an ability to imagine, we shall find ourselves leaving the dark forest bearing gifts.

In conclusion, it is because it is a celebration of relationship that drama therapy is involved with ideas of ultimate truth. This is the god of 'I' and 'Thou', making himself (herself) known in encounter. Because drama, and drama therapy, are specifically aimed at exploring between-ness, they may be seen as religious processes. That is, religion is implicit in the structure, even if not explicit in the subject matter. Ritual and drama originate in a single purpose, that of revealing the meaning and power of life which is interchanged — the gift repaid a thousandfold, the sacrifice leading to rebirth. Whether it be from the ancient doctrine of *katharsis*, which sees theatre as redemption-by-sharing, or the process of personal transformation-by-identification which lies at the heart of religious ritual, drama therapy inherits a concern for the ultimate, and draws its healing power from this fact.

There is no necessity to find a name for this. Indeed, we will discover it assuming another name, and taking on a different significance, every time it is invoked. For it is our truth with one another, and theirs with us; and yet it is neither we nor they, nor is it the combination of both. It is impossible to say precisely what, or who, it is. Perhaps it is naive to try. We can describe the circumstances, but not what actually happens. The closest we can get is to describe it as a *movement* and a *presence*; a movement among us and a presence between us, reconciling us to one another and ourselves, not crowding us, giving us the space we must have to draw closer, touching our finger-tips, looking deep into our eyes before moving on and away. This is how it always is, wherever the drama comes, and we let our imaginations go. In the improvised drama therapy area or on the stage at the Old Vic, in the hospital chapel or the amphitheatre at Epidaurus, we gaze across at one another, waiting for it to begin.

Notes

1. cf Navone (1969), Scholes-Kellogg (1969), Sarbin (1986).
2. 'The choral songs and rites in attribution of the god —associated with the renewal of vegetation, the renewal of the moon, the renewal of the sun, the renewal of the soul, represent the beginning of the Attic tragedy' (J. Campbell, *The Hero With a Thousand Faces*, Paladin, 1988, p143).
3. Indian tradition goes beyond merely claiming a divine origin for the drama, actually endowing the theatre with a genuine scriptural foundation: Bharata's 'Book of the Drama', the *Natyashastra*, dating from the 4th Century AD, is no mere pious actor's vade-mecum, but a work of true religious authority, which became the first of several profound studies of the deeper meaning and spiritual significance of Sanskrit drama.
4. Goffman, *Frame Analysis*, Harper and Row, 1974.
5. 'A complete scheme rite of passage theoretically includes pre-liminal rites (rites of separation), liminal rites (rites of transition) and post-liminal rites (rites of incorporation)'; A Van Gennep, *The Rites of Passage*, Routledge, 1960:10. 'The complete rite is both an initiation into a new condition of being, and a celebration of unity with all who are in that condition' (R. Grainger, *Staging Posts*, Merlin, p.10).

6. Campbell, 1988: 90

7. 'Symbols…operate like a healing draught and divert the fatal incursion of the living Godhead into the hallowed spaces of the church' – C.G. Jung, *The Integration of the Personality*, Kegan Paul, 1940: 59. I have described a similar process with regard to symbols of bereavement in my book *The Message of the Rite*, Lutterworth, 1988: 28–32.

8. Alida Gersie, *Storymaking in Education and Therapy*, Jessica Kingsley Publishers, 1990.

9. J. Campbell, Op. cit. p.22, C.G. Jung refers to 'forms or images of a collective nature, which occur practically all over the earth as constituents of myths and at the same time as autochthonous, individual products of unconscious origin' (C.G. Jung, *Psychology and Religion*, Yale, 1938: 63).

10. This is particularly important when we are considering the relationship between codes of meaning which rely upon rite and myth, and the thought-worlds of psychology and sociology (or, for that matter, systematic theology). Religious rituals cannot really be used to correct social discontinuities or breakdowns in the structure of personal relationships in any way that is directly instrumental. They are not techniques, any more than drama therapy is a technique (cf. Malinowski, 1974).

11. James Roose-Evans, an Anglican priest who is an internationally respected director, is a leader in the field of 'soul journeying' (cf his book '*Inner Journey, Outer Journey*', Ryder, 1987). S. Elizabeth Rees of Turvey Abbey, Bedfordshire, is involved in liturgical drama therapy and runs a 'Summer School in Liturgy and the Arts' in association with Dr Sue Jennings. The imaginative scope of drama therapy is shown by the titles of the lectures and workshops of the British Association of Dramatherapists' National Conference at Manchester in 1989. See Appendix III; also Grainger, (1987, 1988).

Appendix I

The Use of Drama Therapy in the Treatment of Thought Disorder

A grid test was used to measure thought disorder in an unselected group of patients at a psychiatric day hospital, before and after taking part in a course of 10 one-hour sessions of drama therapy. Comparison of results showed a significant treatment effect in the direction of thinking that was more ordered on the part of those subjects whose construing had previously been least intense and consistent.

Introduction

Ordinary life may confirm the network of ideas we have about the world, or prove part of it wrong, in which case the whole has to be readjusted. If this happens too often we may become unwilling, and finally unable, to draw conclusions at all (Bannister, 1963, 1965). The 'construct system' which we use to make sense of what is happening to us now, and to predict what is likely to happen to us in the future, has itself become loosely organised, and represents a vague world in which nothing is either certain or surprising. Examination of the experience and behaviour of thought-disordered patients suggests that their construct systems are of this kind.

Drama involves participation in a highly differentiated inter-personal experience, in which opposing realities must be held in relation, and validation of the experience as a trustworthy way of interpreting and anticipating events. Because of the peculiar power of drama to involve and distance at the same time, leading to an experience of learning about life in depth but without threat, it was suggested that drama therapy might actually have a tightening effect upon loose construct systems. Drama therapy aims at providing an environment which is emotionally secure and structurally recognisable, in which role relationships are clearly defined and epistemological categories easily distinguished. It has been assumed that thought-disordered patients will find this approach aversive – the complex inter-personal reality too confusing, the emotional demands too great (Langley, 1983). We have found that on the contrary cognitive clarity is communicable through dramatic experience, which is not any kind of imitation of life but a participation in the essential processes of human experience, and a way of exposing the relationship between self and other upon which flexibility and definition of thought depend (Wilshire, 1982).

Accounts of the therapeutic effects of drama therapy tend to be somewhat vague, often couched in psychoanalytic language about the achievement of catharsis and the integration of repressed material within consciousness, effects which are notoriously difficult to quantify. The use of drama to increase people's ability to give cognitive structure to their perception of other people suggests the use of techniques which produce results which may be more readily evaluated. Such an approach would serve to validate certain aspects of the private language of schizoid thinking which call forth a response from other people and result in genuine communication. Whether schizoid thinking is characterised as excessively narrow, limited and concrete, or as too broad, generalised and over-inclusive there seems to be general agreement that thought disordered people have difficulties in distinguishing those boundaries of self and other which determine human relationships. There is difficulty in discriminating between subject and object, self-as-participant and self-as-observer, and in categorising different degrees of involvement and concern. What is needed is an opportunity for human experiences of an unambiguous kind, structures simple enough for the thought-disordered to use as matrices for relationship without engulfment, and flexible enough to permit a degree of adventurous experimenting with personal thoughts and feelings.

What follows is an investigation into the kind of thought disorder often associated with schizophrenia, but by no means exclusive to its clinical form. None of the people who acted as subjects had received a clear diagnosis of schizophrenia. All were given the *Bannister and Fransella Grid Test of Thought Disorder* (1966). Those who scored the lowest (i.e. showed most disorder) were studied in greater depth, by means of orthodox case histories. It was these people in whom we were most interested. Had drama therapy clarified their thinking at all?

The field of enquiry remained an open one. Almost all the studies of drama therapy are content to expound the underlying theory and describe what takes place during sessions without venturing into the more hazardous area of evaluating results, (vde. Mazer 1982; Johnson 1982; Landy 1982; Emunah 1983; Rayner 1984; see also Schattner and Courtney 1981, and Langley 1983). An exception is an assessment of drama therapy in a child guidance setting carried out in 1972 by Irwin, Levy and Shapiro, which used a projective test, the Rorschach Index of Repressive Style, and measures of linguistic ability to evaluate the effect of a programme of drama therapy on latency age boys (an RIRS score indicates the extent to which images, emotions and past experiences are verbally labelled and thus available in consciousness in communicable terms). The results indicated that 'dramatherapy was an effective therapeutic technique', significantly lessening repression and increasing verbal fluency. On the other hand, when Spencer, Gillespie and Ekisa (1982) used members of a drama therapy programme as a control group for an investigation into the effectiveness of social-skills training according to a behaviour modification model, only the social-skills training resulted in significant improvement. Subjects in this case were chronic schizophrenics, all of whom had been patients in a psychiatric hospital for several years. The aim of the treatment programme was to improve their 'conversation skills', which the social-skills training did quite effectively.

Believing that drama therapy has more to do with organising thoughts than extending people's conversational repertoire, a colleague, Mary Duggan, and I carried out an investigation in a psychiatric day hospital which made use of personal construct theory to provide a way of evaluating drama therapy. The work of Bannister and his associates suggests the suitability of personal construct theory for the interpretative task. We were concerned to discover whether consistent validation of metaphorical 'as if' constructs concerned with imaginative participation in another person's experience would lead to a more integrated and flexible system for making predictions about other people. Although we used the Grid Test we were not concerned to arrive at clinical diagnosis of thought disorder but to investigate the possibility of degrees of movement in the direction of greater organisation of thinking on the part of those in our sample who were more disordered in their thought. There was always the possibility that these people might find the experience of drama therapy confusing or distracting and become less organised than they had been. In the light of Kelly's suggestion that artistic experience tends to have a 'dilating' effect, making people more relaxed and opening them to new ideas, alternative interpretations of reality (1955: 822), this seemed a real possibility. However, we thought it likely that the experiences we were exploring were of a kind that would contribute to the formation of newer, firmer structures of person-perception and not have a loosening effect. Our experimental hypothesis then was that drama therapy would tighten loose construct formation in thought-disordered people.

Method

Subjects

The programme was included in the therapeutic services provided by a day hospital, care being taken not to present it as any kind of 'experiment'. There was no attempt to select people diagnosed as thought-disordered. Twenty-four subjects were included (17 female and seven male), ranging in age between 38 and 75, each of whom had attained a score of over eight on the vocabulary subscale of the Wechsler Adult Intelligence Scale. Selection was by successive referral: new patients arriving at the hospital were assigned to one of two treatment groups on a 'first come, first served' basis. (This reflects the policy of the day hospital, and also accords well with drama therapy, which requires a good 'mix' of personalities and an unclinical atmosphere of spontaneity.) A pilot study investigating the effect of a ten-week course of drama therapy on seven subjects, two men and five women, taken at random from the Day Hospital population was carried out before proceeding to the main study. The purpose of this was to look for procedural difficulties, both in the administration of the tests, and in the actual drama therapy sessions. The exercise was very useful and led to a certain amount of re-organisation of material and the introduction of new ideas, some of which had not been tried out before.

Procedure

In the main study, both groups of subjects received a course of drama therapy consisting of ten one-hour sessions taking place once a week. These dealt with various aspects of inter-personal activity starting with simple exercises in awareness of others, and became progressively more complex and demanding as they required a greater ability to predict other people's behaviour and share their feelings.

Design

A 'cross-over' design was adopted for the main experiment. During the first ten weeks Group 'A' received treatment, but not Group 'B'; during the second ten weeks, Group 'B' but not Group 'A'. All subjects were tested three times: to begin with, and before and after the second group's sessions. (In this way everybody involved received the benefit of the treatment, and delayed or transitory effects could be noted).

Measures

A change in the direction of increased intensity and consistency of construing was predicted, as measured by the *Thought Disorder Test* (Bannister and Fransella, 1966). Two scores are obtained, and these taken in conjunction yield a thought disorder score expressed in terms of the percentages of non-thought disordered subject scoring lower (Appendix II). The procedure for administering this is described in Appendix II.

The results showed a general improvement in intensity and consistency across both groups of subjects. Fig. 1 shows the difference between mean scores for Experimental and Control conditions.

Figure 1 - Difference between mean scores
for Experimental and Control Conditions

	Intensity		Consistency	
	Exp	*Cont.*	*Exp.*	*Cont.*
Group A	3.54	-0.38	0.03	0.1
Group B	1.50	2.34	0.03	0.1

Figure 2 - Mean scores for Low-Scoring Groups

	Intensity		Consistency	
	Before	*After*	*Before*	*After*
red = Group A	6.87	9.83	0.40	0.73
blue = Group B	7.14	10.94	0.55	0.64

The results were divided into a higher and lower scoring group, the latter consisting of those Ss considered to be thought-disordered to begin with. There was a significant (5% level) improvement in both intensity and consistency for this lower scoring group, who could now be said to be construing in a tighter and more consistent way (as was apparent from their contribution to the drama therapy group). There seems little doubt that intensity and consistency of construing is improved while treatment continues and that the effect persists for some weeks afterwards. Because one group's control condition took place before intervention and the other's after intervention, a simple comparison of combined experimental conditions with combined control conditions is somewhat misleading. In Fig. 2 mean post- and pre-intervention scores of the two groups were compared separately.

It can be seen that each group's experimental score is higher both than its own and the other group's pre-intervention scores. When the group is divided up according to whether the control condition preceded or followed the experimental one, Group B (control-experimental) shows a definite improvement during the experimental condition, and Group A (experimental-control) a slight fall-off during the retrospective control condition. However, of the seven people who scored less than ten[1] for intensity at the beginning of the investigation, all showed improved scores at the end, three having lifted well clear of the thought disorder criterion by the third testing. Of the eight scoring less than ten at the start of the actual drama therapy sessions, seven had increased their scores by the end, the eighth showing less of an increase than during the control period, but still scoring higher than she had done to begin with.

Discussion

(1) As predicted, a degree of improvement was obtained in the patients' construing of other people following drama therapy. However, the marked trend in Group B towards improved performance during the pre-intervention period indicates that Day Hospital attendance contributed to this finding. It would seem that drama therapy may, therefore, enhance existing benefits of attendance, although a truly untreated control group would be required to give this interpretation more substance. The results from Group B reveal the sudden invalidation of part of an individual's construct system within the course of a single testing, which is associated with clinical depression (Bannister 1960). Although this only occurred in one out of a group of twelve subjects, the statistical effect is dramatic.

(2) The experiment underlined the difficulties involved in trying to be experimentally rigorous in a setting in which rigid control of subjects can be counter-productive, particularly when dealing with a treatment modality which puts a high premium on spontaneity and freedom of expression (Grainger, 1985). Each of the participants was informed that he or she could decline to participate at any stage of the programme and there was no attempt to subject them to any kind of selection process. The necessity of administering the Thought Disorder Test tended to give an unwelcome clinical flavour to the proceedings, and consequently some of the exercises were designed to produce results which could be compared and assimilated as part of the drama therapy sessions. For example an informal repertory grid was built into the exercise comprising the first and last sessions of each programme. Group 'A' refused to allow themselves to be scored, but Group 'B' produced a mean group intensity score of 178 at the last session, compared with 162 at the first one.

> In the sessions of drama therapy described here, we worked with individuals through the group medium. In drama therapy men and women were encouraged to reveal their uniqueness in a setting designed specifically to allow a comparison of similarities and differences, one in which the presence of

structure serves the purpose of identifying the possibility of freedom – that is, the range of forms which may be taken by action and inter-action that is *free*. In practical terms this meant that the integrity of the course of sessions must be preserved without the introduction of evaluative devices from outside. As we found to our cost, there is no way in which formal measures disguised as drama therapy exercises may be passed off as anything other than what they are – reductionist attempts to harness spontaneity and use it for purposes alien to itself. This is not to say that the experience of drama therapy produces an effect aversive to psychological testing, but only that the state of mind associated with drama therapy refuses to compromise with formal instruction if this is imposed on it *in situ*, that is, actually during the course of a session. Attempts designed to measure the effect of a single exercise in a session are almost invariably doomed to failure – group members either lose the thread of what is going on in the session as a whole, or they simply refuse to try and make the transition from one way of thinking to another. Instrumental thinking, the kind used for solving problems in the 'real' world, must wait until the session is over. For the present, a more intuitive approach holds sway.

(3) The evidence presented here suggests that the ability to think clearly and practically is in no way lessened by these excursions into drama.[2] Certainly, in terms of expressive behaviour, all of the people in this investigation who appeared to be construing most loosely participated more creatively at the end of the course than they had done to begin with. As far as their ability to think purposefully towards the performance of a set task – that is, making consistent sense of the relationship between the various elements and constructs of the Grid Test of Thought Disorder – all twelve showed a degree of improvement. Four of these people have been examined in greater depth in the text of Chapter 6.

(4) To conclude: The investigation described above would certainly have benefited from using more subjects, but interesting effects reveal themselves within individual grids, even when the overall statistical significance is not apparent, and it would be a pity to risk 'throwing out the baby with the bath water' by trying to be too rigorous in applying scientific controls, and so inhibiting the behaviour to be studied. In this case the use of the Thought Disorder Test seems particularly appropriate because it deals explicitly with the way people present themselves to, and are construed by others, and the test task (of sorting photographs and judging facial expressions) leads more or less naturally into exercises in personal interaction and relationship. Certainly, the experiment may be said to have contributed to a very real improvement in patients' health brought about by the overall Day Hospital Programme.

(5) Taken as a whole, the results show a more striking increase in intensity than consistency. Group B, in fact, scored higher during the control period than the experimental. This result was not expected, of course; all the same it should be said that it accords well with the way in which people involved in artistic pursuits are observed to behave – which is not less effectively but certainly less predictably than the norm. When subjects have been systematically encouraged to be inventive and to find new ways of 'putting things together', consistency may not appear so important as originality. It has been demonstrated that this kind of exploratory behaviour has the effect of improving people's competence in organising their behaviour, whether this be expressive or instrumental (Eisner, 1985). It would seem to follow that they are also made more skilful at *re*-organising it. Were our subjects encouraged by the drama therapy exercises to experiment with new ways of making relationships between elements?

(6) Because of the particular terms of reference of our study, there was considerable variation among individuals with regard to the 'looseness – tightness' dimension of construing, with scores ranging from 2.83 to 21.41 for Intensity. It is interesting to note that the only subjects to score lower after treatment than before occur above the 'cut-off mark' for low scorers (I., C.F). All those at the lower end of the scale scored higher after drama therapy than before, i.e. six subjects, plus three from the Pilot Study. This suggests that drama therapy is effective as a way of tightening those construct systems that tend toward looseness. It may have other therapeutic effects, of course (including the 'dilating' effect mentioned by Kelly in cases where construing is over-tight). However, it is this effect that interests us here, as it seems to provide evidence of the integrating effect of drama upon fragmented human awareness. Perhaps the way is now open for an investigation which would involve people diagnosed as thought-disordered schizophrenics.

Notes

1. Original Grid Test score = 1000
2. Eliot Eisner claims that open ended activity of the creative/exploratory kind involved in drama therapy actually improves people's competence in organising behaviour, whether it be expressive, or instrumental (1985).

References

Bannister, D. (1960), 'Conceptual Structure in Thought-Disorder Schizophrenia', *Journal of Mental Science*, 106, 1230–1249.

Bannister, D. (1963), 'The Genesis of Schizophrenic Thought Disorder: a Serial Invalidation Hypothesis', *Brit. J. Psych.*, 109, 680–686.

Bannister, D. (1965), 'The Genesis of Schizophrenic Thought Disorder: re-test of the Serial Invalidation Hypothesis', *Brit. J. Psych.*, III, 327–372.

Bannister, D. (1966), 'A Grid Test of Schizophrenic Thought Disorder', *Brit. J. Soc. & Clin. Psychol.*, 5, 95–102.

Bannister, D. & Fransella, F. (1986), *Inquiring Man*, Croom Helm, London.

Eisner, E. W. (1985), *The Art of Educational Evaluation*, Falmer.

Emunah, R. (1983), 'Dramatherapy with Adult Psychiatric Patients', *Arts in Psychotherapy*, 10, 77–84.

Grainger, R. (1985), 'Using Drama Creatively in Therapy', *Dramatherapy*, 8, 2, 33–46.

Irwin, C., Levy, P. & Shapiro, M. (1972), 'Assessment of Dramatherapy in a Child Guidance Setting', *Group Psychotherapy and Psychodrama*, 25, 3, 105–116.

Johnson, D. R. (1982), 'Developmental Approaches in Drama Therapy', *Arts in Psychotherapy*, 9, 183–9.

Kelly, G. (1963), *A Theory of Personality*, Norton, New York.

Landy, R. J. (1982), 'Training the Drama Therapist: a Four Part Model', *Arts in Psychotherapy*, 9, 91–99.

Langley, D. M. (1983), *Dramatherapy and Psychiatry*, Croom Helm, London.

Mazer, R. (1982), 'Drama Therapy for the Elderly in a Day Centre', *Hospital and Community Psychiatry*, 33, 7, 577–579.

Rayner, P. (1984), 'Psychodrama as a Medium for Intermediate Treatment', *Br. J. Social Work*, 7, 4.

Schattner, G. & Courtney, R., (Eds), (1981), *Drama in Therapy*, vol. II, Drama Book Specialists, New York.

Spencer, P. G., Gillespie, C.R. & Ekisa, E.G. (1983), 'A Controlled Comparison of the Effects of Social Skills Training and Remedial Drama on the Conversational Skills of Chronic Schizophrenic Inpatients', *Brit. J. Psych.*, 143, 165–172.

Wilshire, B. (1982), *Role Playing and Identity*, Indiana University Press, Bloomington.

Instructions for administering the Grid Test for Thought Disorder

Place in front of the subject an array of eight photographs, four male and four female. Ask the subject to study these, and tell him he will be asked questions about the people in them. Ask him which of them is most likely to be KIND. When he has made his choice, write the letter (A-H) printed on the back on the score sheet under the heading KIND. Ask the subject to choose the person most likely to be KIND from the seven remaining photographs. Note the letter on the back on the score sheet under his first choice, in the KIND rank. Continue until he has ranked all eight photographs, from most KIND to least. The photographs are shuffled and the procedure repeated, the subject being asked now to rank STUPID. Proceed in this way until he has rank ordered all eight photographs on six constructs – KIND, STUPID, SELFISH, SINCERE, MEAN, and HONEST. Finally, give the subject the following instructions: 'Now I should like you to do it all again. Change your mind if you want to – it's not a memory test, and there's no right or wrong way of doing it. I just want to know how you feel about these people now you've thought about it.' Repeat the test procedure as before, to produce two sets of ranked letters forming two grids.

Diagrammatic summary of the results of a grid-test to measure thought disorder.

K = Kind **St** = Stupid **Se** = Selfish **Si** = Sincere **M** = Mean **H** = Honest
A = Before treatment **B** = After treatment *(each test contains two grids)*

Principle Constructs	**Related Constructs**	**Significant Correlations**
K	Si	.88

(In all cases, Principle Constructs are shown in the top line and Related Constructs in the bottom.)

TM *A: Intensity 7.76: Consistency .70*

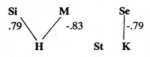 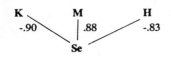 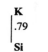

B: Intensity 12.95: Consistency .85

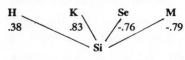 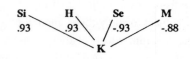

JP *A: Intensity 5.16: Consistency .29*

St Si K H Se M   Se K H Si St M

B: Intensity 7.41: Consistency .75

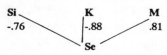 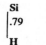

EG *A: Intensity 9.67: Consistency .68*

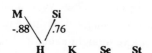

M Si K H St Se   H K Se St

B: Intensity 12.87: Consistency .68

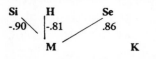 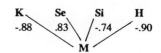

DT *A: Intensity 5.22: Consistency .20*

H
.81
Si M St K   H Se K St Si

B: Intensity 7.41: Consistency -.03

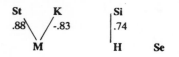 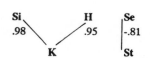

Programme of the British Association of Dramatherapists' National Conference, Manchester, 1989

'A Creation Myth' (Pat Walls); 'Exploring Body Image' (Shirley Casson); 'Dramatherapy and Eating Disorders' (Sue Jennings); 'The Shape of Feeling: image shape and sound in expressing feelings' (David Brailsford); 'Living Soap – the power of soap operas in our lives' (Tone Harwood); 'A Ceremony for the Tropical Rain Forests' (Steve Mitchell); 'Guided Fantasy and the Mind/Body Link' (Peter Phillippson); 'Acting Ourselves: Character and Body Language in Reichian Therapy' (Nick Totton); 'Natural Self-Expression through Dance' (Merle Van Den Bosch); 'The Body of Dramatherapy Knowledge' (Helen Payne); 'Images and Archetypes of the Tarot' (Madeline Anderson-Warren); 'Body and Image in Shakespeare' (Marina Jenkyns); 'The Effects of Childhood Sexual Abuse on Body and Image' (Anne Bannister); 'The Psychodrama Director; Image and Performance' (Don Feasey); 'Biofeedback' (John Willen); 'Images of Oppression' (Gordon Wiseman); 'Exploring Addiction through Dramatherapy' (Laura Atkinson and Louise Larkinson); 'Aids: Taboo or Not Taboo' (Mike Fitzsimmons); 'Primal Dance' (Merle Van Den Bosch); 'Look at me, I'm Flowing. The Images of T'ai Chi' (Linda Chase Broda); 'Personagrams – group sculpting' (Sue Mitchell); 'Bodies in Space' (David Powley); 'A Journey Round our Body' (Dorothy Langley); 'Metaphor in Therapy', (Roy Shuttleworth); 'Images of Oppression' (Gordon Wiseman); 'The Body Politic' (David Powley); 'Getting My Own Back – Exploring Sexual Abuse' (David Pithers).

The theme of the conference was 'Body and Image in Dramatherapy'.

Bibliography

Artaud, A. *Le Théatre et son Double*, trans. M. C. Richards, Evergreen, 1966.

Bannister, D. 'Conceptual Structure in Thought-Disorder Schizophrenia' *J. Mental Science*, 106, 1230–1249, 1960.

'Personal Construct Theory; a summary and experimental paradigm' *Acta Psychol.*, 20, 104–120, 1962a.

'The Nature and Measurement of Schizophrenic Thought Disorder', *J. Mental Science*, 108, 824–42, 1962b.

'The Genesis of Schizophrenic Thought Disorder; a Serial Invalidation Hypothesis', *Brit. J. Psych.* 109, 680–686, 1963.

'The Genesis of Schizophrenic Thought Disorder; re-test of the Serial Invalidation Hypothesis' *Brit. J. Psych.* III, 327–372, 1965.

'The Nonsense of Effectiveness', *New Forum; the Journal of the Psychiatry & Psychology Association*, August 13, 1980.

Bannister, D., Adams-Webber, J. R., Penn, W. I., & Radley, A. R. 'Reversing the Process of Thought Disorder: A Serial Validation Experiment', *Brit. J. Soc. & Clin. Psychol.* 14, 169–180, 1975.

Bannister, D. & Fransella, F. 'A Grid-Test of Schizophrenic Thought Disorder', *Brit. J. Soc. & Clin. Psychol.*, 5, 95–102, 1966.

Inquiring Man, Croom Helm, 1986.

Bannister, D. & Salmon, P. 'Schizophrenic Thought Disorder: Specific or Diffuse?', *Brit. J. Med. Psychol.* 35, 215–219, 1966.

Bateson, G. *Steps to an Ecology of Mind*, Paladin, 1973.

Bateson, G., Jackson, D., Haley, J. & Weakland, J. 'Towards a Theory of Schizophrenia', *Behavioural Science*, 1, 251–264, 1956.

'A Method for Distinguishing and Evaluating Formal Thinking Disorders in Schizophrenia', in J. S. Kasanin (Ed.), *Language and Thought in Schizophrenia*, Norton, 1944.

Beck, A. T., Ward, C. H., Mendelson, M., Mock, J. & Erbaugh, J. 'An Inventory for Measuring Depression', *Arch. of Gen. Psychiat.*, 4, 561–567, 1961.

Brooke, P. *The Empty Space*, MacGibbon and Kee, 1968.

Buber, M. *Pointing the Way*, RKP, 1957.

I and Thou, RKP, 1958.

Burns, E. *Theatricality: A Study of Conventionality in the Theatre and in Social Life*, Harper & Row, 1972.

Butcher, S. H. *A Commentary on Aristotle's 'Poetics'* (1894), Dover, 1951.

Cameron, N. 'Experimental Analysis of Schizophrenic Thinking' in J. Kasanin (Ed.) *Language and Thought in Schizophrenia*, Norton, 1944.

Campbell, J. *The Hero With a Thousand Faces*, Paladin, 1988.

Casson, J. 'Shamanistic Elements of Oriental Theatre with Special Reference to the Traditional Forms of Drama in Sri Lanka.' (unpub. M. A. thesis, Birmingham University, 1978).

Cheshire, N. M. *The Nature of Psychodynamic Interpretation*, Wiley, 1975.

Cox, M. *Structuring the Therapeutic Process*, amended edition, Jessica Kingsley Publishers, 1988.

Durkheim, E. & Mauss, M. *Primitive Classification*, (trans. R. Needham), RKP, 1963.

Eisner, E. W. *The Art of Educational Evaluation*, Falmer Press, 1985.

Eliade, M. *Patterns in Comparative Religion*, Sheed & Ward, 1958.

Myths, Dreams and Mysteries, Collins, 1968.

Erikson, E. *Childhood and Society*, Penguin, 1965.

Toys and Reasons, Boyars, 1977.

Fromm, E. *Fear of Freedom*, RKP, 1960.

Gennep, A. Van. *The Rites of Passage* (Trans. M. B. Vizedom & G. L. Caffee), RKP, 1960.

Gersie, A., *Storymaking in Education and Therapy*, Jessica Kingsley Publishers, 1990.

Goffman, E. *The Presentation of Self in Everyday Life*, Penguin, 1971.

Grainger, R. *Watching for Wings*, Darton, Longman & Todd, 1979.

'Using Drama Creatively in Therapy', *Dramatherapy*, 8, 2, 33–46, 1985.

Staging Posts, Merlin, 1977

The Message of the Rite, Lutterworth, 1988.

Harré, R. & Seccord, P. F. *The Explanation of Social Behaviour*, Blackwell, 1972.

Heidegger, M. *Being and Time*, Blackwell, 1962.

Jennings, S., *Dramatherapy with Families and Groups: Waiting in the Wings*, Jessica Kingsley Publishers, 1990.

Jennings, S. 'The Impact of the Body in Non-Verbal Methods of Therapy', in S. Jennings, *Creative Therapy*, Kemble Press, 1983.

Jung, C. G. *Psychology and Religion*, (trans. H. G. & C. E. Baynes), Yale, 1938.

The Integration of the Personality, Kegan Paul, 1940.

Psychology and Alchemy, Collective Works, RKP, 1953.

'On the Relation of Analytical Psychology to Poetic Art', *Contributions to Analytical Psychology*, (trans. H. G. & C. E. Baynes), London, 1928.

Johnson, D. R. 'Drama Therapy and the Schizoid Condition', in G. Schattner & R. Courtney, (Eds), *Drama in Therapy*, vol. 2, Drama Book Specialists, 1981.

Jones, H. 'Creativity and Depression', in Epting, F. & Landfield, A. W. (Eds.), *Anticipating Personal Construct Psychology*, Univ. of Nebraska Press, 1985.

Kelly, G. A. *The Psychology of Personal Constructs*, Norton, 1955

'In Whom Confide; On Whom Depend for What?', *4th Memorial Lecture*, New York Soc. Clinical Psychologists, Dec.7, 1962.

Laing, R. D. & Esterson, A. *Sanity, Madness and the Family*, Penguin, 1970.

Laing, R. D. 'The Spiral of Perspectives', *New Society*, Nov. 10, 713–716, 1966.

Landy, R. *Dramatherapy: Concepts and Practice*. Thomas, 1986.

Langer, S. *Philosophy in a New Key*, Oxford University Press, 1951.

Langley, D. M. *Dramatherapy and Psychiatry*, Croom-Helm, 1983.

Lidz, T. *The Family and Human Adaptation*, Hogarth, 1964.

'The Family, Language, and the Transmission of Schizophrenia', in D. Rosenthal and S. Kety (Eds.), *The Transmission of Schizophrenia*, Pergamon, 1968.

The Origin and Treatment of Schizophrenic Disorders, Hutchinson, 1975.

Maher, B. *Clinical Psychology & Personality: The Selected Papers of George Kelly*, R. Krieger Pub., Huntington, N. Y., 1979.

Malinowski, B. *Magic, Science & Religion*, Souvenir Press, 1974.

May, R. *The Courage to Create*, Collins, 1975.

Merleau-Ponty, M. *The Phenomenology of Perception*, Routledge, 1962.

Moreno, J. L. *Psychodrama*, Vol. I, Beacon House, 1972.

Navone, J. *Towards a Theology of Story*, Paulist Press, 1977.

Polanyi, M. *Personal Knowledge*, Routledge, 1958.

Ross, M. V. 'Depression, Self-Concept and Personal Constructs', in Epting, F. & Landfield, A. W., *Anticipating Personal Construct Psychology*, Univ. of Nebraska Press, 1985.

Rowe, D. 'Depression is a Prison', in Epting, F. & Landfield, A. W., *Anticipating Personal Construct Psychology*, Univ. of Nebraska Press, 1985.

Sarbin, T. S. (Ed.) *Narrative Psychology*, Praeger, 1986.

Schattner, G. A. & Courtney, R., (Eds), *Drama in Therapy*, vols 1 and 2, Drama Book Specialists, 1981.

Schaff, T. J. *Catharsis in Drama, Healing and Ritual*, Univ. of California, 1980.

Scholes-Kellogg, *The Nature of Narrative*, OUP, 1969.

Smail, D. J. *Psychotherapy, A Personal Approach*, Dent, 1978.

Spolin, V. *Theatre Game File*, CEMREL, 1975.

'Theatre Games', in G. Schattner and R. Courtney (Eds.) *Drama in Therapy*, Vol. 2, Drama Book Specialists, 1981.

Stanislavski, C. *An Actor Prepares*, Theatre Arts, 1936.

Storr, A. *The Dynamics of Creation*, Penguin, 1972.

The Art of Psychotherapy, Secker & Warburg/Heinemann, 1979.

Sullivan, H. S. 'The Language of Schizophrenia', in J. S. Kasanin (Ed.) *Language and Thought in Schizophrenia*, Norton, 1944.

Schizophrenia as a Human Process, Norton, 1974.

Wilshire, B. *Role Playing and Identity*, Indiana University Press, 1982.

Winnicott, D. W. *Playing and Reality*, Tavistock, 1971.

Wynne, L. & Singer, M. 'Thought Disorder, Family Relations of Schizophrenics. 1: A Research Strategy'. *Arch. Gen. Psychiat.* 9: 191–198, 1963a.

'Thought Disorder, Family Relations of Schizophrenics. 2: A Classification of Forms of Thinking'. *Arch. Gen. Psychiat.* 9: 199–206, 1963b.

Suggested Reading

Achterberg, J. *Imagery in Healing*, New Science, 1985.

Artaud, A. *Le Théâtre et son Double*, Evergreen, 1966.

Bannister, D. & Fransella, F. *Inquiring Man*, Croom-Helm, 1986.

Butcher, S. H. *A Commentary on Aristotle's Poetics*, Dover, 1951.

Cox, M. *Structuring the Therapeutic Process*, amended edition, Jessica Kingsley Publishers, 1988
  Coding the Therapeutic Process, amended edition, Jessica Kingsley Publishers, 1988

Jennings, S. (Ed) *Creative Therapy*, Kemble Press, 1983.
  Dramatherapy, Theory and Practice for Teachers and Clinicians, Croom Helm, 1987.

Kelly, G. *A Theory of Personality: The Psychology of Personal Constructs*, Norton, 1963.

May, R. *The Courage to Create*, Collins, 1975.

Moreno, J. L. *Psychodrama*, Vol. I, Beacon House, 1972.

Schattner, G. & Courtney, R., (Eds), *Drama in Therapy*, Vols. 1 & 2, Drama Book Specialists, 1981.

Wilshire, B. *Role Playing & Identity*, Indiana University Press, 1982.

Winnicott, D. W. *Playing and Reality*, Tavistock, 1971.

Glossary

Abreaction: Reduction of emotional distress by the release of disturbed behaviour, which is unconsciously determined and reflects previous unresolved conflicts.

Aesthetic distance: The interposition of an idea or an artefact between a perceiving subject and the object of his/her perception, with the result that intensity of perception is increased by the effort involved in overcoming the obstacle. In the theatre this effect is produced by the actual physical separation of audience from stage.

Archetype: Images fundamental of truth affecting the entire human race at unconscious level, and expressing themselves in dreams and the cross-cultural symbolism of art.

Katharsis: The purging of the effects of a pent-up emotion by bringing them to the surface of consciousness.

Object Relations Theory: An explanation of the human experience of relationship in terms of the development of infantile fantasy to take account of the mother as a separate person (sometimes called symbiosis and individuation.)

Personal Construct Theory: A theory of personal and social psychology devised by George Kelly, centring around the idea of 'constructive alternativism' according to which the individual is free to experiment with alternative ways of making sense of (construing) what happens to him/her in order to predict and control events.

Psychodrama: Form of group therapy involving the dramatic staging of a patient's signs and symptoms or problems, by fellow members ('alternative egos') and members of the therapeutic team.

Repertory Grid: Instrument used by Personal Construct psychologists to explore attitudes and feelings. In the grid, categories (constructs) and people (elements) inter-relate to produce a picture of the way someone organises his or her personal world (construct system).

Rite of Passage: Corporate religious ceremonial representing and implementing an important change in social and religious status which affects a particular individual or group, and also the wider group to which they belong.

Sculpt: Pose adopted to express an idea, feeling or attitude of mind in the form of a living statue. Sculpting may be carried out alone, using one's own body, in pairs, using someone else's body as the medium or in groups ('group sculpting').

Shaman: Folk-priest of N. Asia and Indian sub-continent, etc., characterized by the ability to journey in trance to the world of those spirits controlling disease and death and liberating the sick from their influence.

Transitional Object: Something occupying an intermediate area of experience between infantile solipsism and acceptance of another person (i.e. the mother) as an independent being: the first 'not-me' possession.

Index

References to notes are indicated by an 'n' after the page reference e.g. '28n'

abreaction 150
'active imagination' 64
actors, depressed 47,
    48–9, 51
aesthetic distance 12,
    17–18, 19–21, 28n,
    30, 150
    and personality 48, 49
    and ritual 123
Ancient Greek theatre 14,
    20–1, 28n, 120
animal psychodrama 86,
    89
anorexia, and depression
    51–2
anxiety 40, 75
    case study 114–16
archetypes 35, 39n, 126,
    150
Aristotle 12, 23
art and reality 17–18,
    28n, 33, 34, 36
Artaud, Antonin 28n, 122

artistic criticism *see*
    therapeutic criticism
artists, depressed 45–7
authorisation 25
'awareness' exercises 78,
    79

Bannister, D. 61, 96, 134
    on depression 40
    on schizophrenia 54, 56,
    57, 58, 62–3, 67n
    see also Thought Disorder
    Test
Bateson, G. 13, 55, 67n
Beck, A. T. 42
bi-polar depression 42
bodily positions 76
    see also sculpting
'body awareness' 50
'body image' 50–1
boundaries between self
    and other 11, 31–2,
    135
British Association of
    Dramatherapists'
    conference 133n, 144
Brooke, Peter 121
Buber, Martin 20, 22, 28n
Burns, E. 19

Campbell, J. 125
case-histories 83–98,
    114–16
Cezanne example 18
child development
    and depression 31, 41,
    43–4

and schizophrenia 30,
    31, 54–6
choral performance,
    ancient Greek 120–21
Christian liturgiologists
    130, 133n
closing a therapy session
    81
collective unconscious 35
concepts, Kelly's view 37
'concrete thinking' 68n
conference, British
    Association of
    Dramatherapists' 133n,
    144
'construct sub-systems' 26
Construct Theory *see*
    Personal Construct
    Theory; Repertory
    Grid; Thought
    Disorder Test
'constructive alternativism'
    26, 36
constructs 37–8, 39n, 41
controversial topic game
    example 107–8
core constructs,
    pre-emptive 41–2, 85,
    93
core roles 23, 42
Cox, M. 56, 60
'creative acceptability' 46
'creative apperception' 17
creativity, and depression
    45–7
'credulous approach' 36,
    83

death fear 32
depression 9, 11–12, 13,
    40–52, 71
  and creativity 45–7
  and Construct Theory
    13, 40–1, 45
  development 31, 41,
    43–4
  under-distancing 48, 49
Dionysus rites 120
disclosure *see* self-disclosure
distance *see* aesthetic
    distance; psychic
    distance
dithyrambs 120
'double bind' hypotheses
    13, 55, 67n
'doubling' techniques 82n
drama therapy aims, 9,
    11–12
dramatherapists 129–30
  conference 133n, 144
Dramaturgical Theory of
    Social Analysis 29n, 64
dream states, and
    imagination 34–5
'DT' case-history 93–6,
    97–8
Duggan, Mary 136

educational drama 12
'EG' case-history 90–3, 97
Eisner, E. W. 100–1, 102,
    141n
Ekisa, E. G. 136
Eliade, M. 35, 124
engulfment (fusion) 22,
    23, 25, 27, 30, 33

Esterton, A. 55, 56–7, 60
evaluation of drama
    therapy 99–117,
    135–41
  example 103–17
'existential validation' 99
experimental theatre 129
extrapersonal relationships
    73, 74

family
  and schizophrenia 54–6
  see also mothering; parents
family sculpts 80–1
  examples 89, 93, 96
fear 23–4
  life and death 32
'Fragmentation Corollary'
    26
Fransella 96
  see also Thought Disorder
    Test
freedom-in-structure 12,
    71, 81, 140
Freud, S. 30, 44
Fromm, Erich 38n, 44, 53
fusion *see* engulfment

games 14, 74–5
Gillespie, C. R. 136
'God within' 126
Goffman, E. 10, 29n, 64
'good-enough mothering'
    31, 43
'grace-yielding
    sacraments' 125

Greek classical theatre 14,
    20–1, 28n, 120
Grid Test for Thought
    Disorder *see* Thought
    Disorder Test

Harré, R. 29
healing rituals, ancient
    120, 121
Heidegger, M. 29n
'heroic journeys' 125, 126
Hindu drama 14, 121,
    132n

'I-Thou'/'I-It'
    relationships 22, 28n,
    132
identification 11, 20, 27,
    38n, 132,
  'secondary' 32
'if'-faculty 11, 65
imagination 20, 31, 34–6,
    130–31
  'active' 64
imaginative play 33, 34
immaturity 44
'impermeable' construct
    systems 97
impersonal relationships
    73, 74
Indian drama 14, 121,
    132n
individuation 22–3, 25–6,
    30
Institute of Drama
    Therapy 129

interpersonal relationships 12, 73–4

intrapersonal relationships 73–4

'irrational living force' 122

Irwin, C. 135–6

Japanese drama 14, 121

Jennings, Sue 50, 130

Johnson, David Read 59–60, 73

journeys 35, 77, 110, 122

'JP' case-study 86–90, 97

Jung, C. G. 35, 39n
  symbolism 125, 126, 133n

katharsis 12, 66, 128, 150
  of ritual 125, 132

Kelly, George 13, 23, 36–8, 45, 62, 64

Laing, R. D. 26, 55, 56–7, 60

Langer, Susan 30

Langley, Dorothy 75, 117

language
  of ritual 126–7
  of schizophrenics 60–1, 63, 135

learned helplessness 52n

Levy, P. 135–6

Lidz, T. 55, 58, 59, 67n

life fear 32

'looseness' of construct systems 10, 38
  and depression 40, 45
  examples 84, 96
  and drama therapy 129, 134, 136, 141
  and schizophrenia 57, 63, 64

manic-depressives 47

maturity 44, 46

May, Rollo 17, 17–18, 22, 32

Mead, G. H. 34

'meaning of life' 119, 126, 128, 130

metaphor 14, 76–7, 101, 117

mimesis 21–2, 23, 28n, 29n

mirroring 79, 107

Moreno, Jakob 81–2n, 99, 117–8n

mothering 39n, 54
  'good enough' 31, 43

Motikoyo, Zeami 121

mountain drama example 112–13

mutual acceptance, in therapy 72

mutual concern, in therapy 73

mystic journeys 35, 77, 110, 122

mystification 13, 55, 56–7

myths 125–6, 133n

names game 79

narrators, in therapy groups 109

newness and healing 124–5

Noh plays 121

obesity, and depression 51–2

Object Relations Theory 12, 30, 31–2, 150
  and schizophrenia 56, 58

objectivity, and evaluation 99–101, 140

observation game 107

obsessional neurosis 96–7

obstacle touching game 109–10

'oral' stage of development 44

'over-distancing' 48

painful feelings 24, 25

parents
  and child's depression 43–4
  and child's schizophrenia 54–6
  see also mothering

participation, importance of 20, 100, 121, 135

perceptual image, and theatre 19, 22

'permeable construct systems' 32

'person blindness' 10–11

Personal Construct Theory
    9–10, 13, 26, 36–8,
    134, 150
  and depression 13,
    40–1, 45
  and drama therapy
    evaluation 135,
    136–41
  and schizophrenia 13,
    54, 57, 58–9, 61,
    62–3
  see also Repertory Grid;
    Thought Disorder Test
personal testimony
    99–100
pity 23–4
playing 33, 34
Playing and Reality 53
Polanyi, Michael 100
pre-emptive core
    constructs 41–2, 85, 93
'presence' 132
private languages 60–1,
    63, 135
psychiatrists 130
psychic distance 30
  see also aesthetic distance
psychodrama 99–100,
    129, 150
  animal 86, 89
psychological distance 28n
psychological integration
    66
psychotherapists 130
psychotherapy
  and depression 42

and drama therapy 99,
    128, 129
and schizophrenia 59

reality 9–10, 11
  and drama 17, 18–20,
    21, 26–7, 28n, 66
  and ritual 124, 125
'receptive' character 44
Rees, Elizabeth 133n
relaxation 74, 77
religion
  and myths 125–6
  see also ritual
Repertory Grid 150
reporting game 79
rites of passage 122, 125,
    127, 132–3n, 151
  drama therapy compared
    124
ritual, religious 14,
    119–28, 129, 131–2
  ancient theatre origins
    120–21
  drama compared 123–4,
    127–8
  language 126–7
  structure 123, 124
roles 14, 29n, 72–4
  examples 88–9, 93
  reversal 14, 73–4, 81–2n
Roose-Evans, James 133n
Rorschach Index of
    Repressive Style 135–6
Rowe, Dorothy 41
Royal Academy of
    Dramatic Art 129–30

scene-setting, for therapy
    14, 71–2
schizogenic families 55
schizophrenia 10–11, 12,
    30, 48, 53–68, 71
  development 54–7
  grid test investigation
    136
  Object Relations Theory
    56, 58
  Personal Construct
    Theory 13, 54, 57,
    58–9, 61, 62–3
scientific objectivity
    99–101, 140
sculpting 14, 76, 79–80,
    151
  examples 86, 89, 92,
    104–5
  family sculpts 80–1, 89,
    93, 96
'secondary identification'
    32
Secord, P. F. 29
security 54, 64, 66
'self', and 'other' 9, 17,
    21, 24
  boundaries 11, 31–2,
    135
  and depression 41, 42,
    46
self-disclosure 78, 83, 117
  example 115–16
self-esteem. and
    depression 43, 49
self-expression 78, 79–80
self-reportage 83
Seligman, M. E. P. 45, 52n

'serial invalidation' 57, 62, 67n

'shadow' archetype 35

Shaman 151

Shamanism 35, 39n, 122, 130

shared characteristic game 79, 108

Shapiro, M. 135–6

sharing 10, 20, 100, 113–14, 132

Singer, M. 56

'skewed' families 13, 55, 67n

'slot-rattling' 41

Smail, D. J. 74, 100

Spencer, P. G. 136

'spiral of perspectives' 26

spiritual wholeness 14, 131

standardised testing 101

Stanislavski, C. 11, 65

Steiner, George 127

stories 119–20, 122, 125–6

Storr, Anthony 42, 44, 45, 53

structure, of drama therapy freedom and 11–12, 71–81, 117, 135

and schizophrenia 58, 64, 65

'subjective object' 32, 39n

symbolism 12–13, 30–8
 archetypes 35
 and ritual 124, 125, 126
 see also transitional objects

testing, standardised 101

therapeutic criticisms 102–3
 example 103–17

Thought Disorder Test 92, 133, 135–41, 143–4
 individual results 85, 91, 92, 96–8, 144

thought disorders *see* schizophrenia, Thought Disorder Test

tightness of construct systems *see* looseness of construct systems

'TM' case-study 83–6, 96–7

'Tony' case-study 114–16

toy theatre example 24–5

'transitional objects' 12–13, 33–4, 129, 151
 and schizophrenia 53, 58, 59

tree perception examples 18

'under-distancing' 48, 49

'universalisation of emotions' 24

validation 10, 118n
 and schizophrenia 13, 63, 64, 67

variability, in construing 40

weight, and depression 51–2

Wilshire, B. 21, 22–3, 25, 26, 28n, 135

Winnicott, D. W. 17, 30, 32, 33, 39n
 'good-enough mothering' 31, 43

transitional objects 12, 53, 58, 59

Wise Person image 77

Wynne, L. 56